No Fear

Shea Mahoney

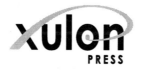

Copyright © 2010 by Shea Mahoney

No Fear
by Shea Mahoney

Printed in the United States of America

ISBN 9781609577889

All rights reserved solely by the author. The author guarantees all contents are original and do not infringe upon the legal rights of any other person or work. No part of this book may be reproduced in any form without the permission of the author. The views expressed in this book are not necessarily those of the publisher. Some names have been changed.

Unless otherwise indicated, Bible quotations are taken from The New King James Version, Copyright © 1997 by Thomas Nelson, Inc. and The New International Version, Copyright © 1973, 1978, 1984 by International Bible Society (Zondervan Publishing House).

www.xulonpress.com

Acknowledgements

Christi,

For your time, your prayers, your efforts, your encouragement, and your friendship, I could never thank you enough. You have been more of a blessing than you could ever know.

Proverbs 27:17

To my family,

Words cannot express what you mean to me. Thank you for your love and your support in everything. I am so blessed to have each of you in my life.

Introduction

When I first felt God's calling to write this book I questioned Him continually. I thought it must be a side-effect of the post-surgery pain medication making me think crazy thoughts. I knew God couldn't be calling me to write a book because I wasn't capable. I knew I didn't have the talent or ability to do this. I never liked English literature or writing, and I definitely didn't like the idea of telling so many people my story, of letting them into the unseen world of my emotions and thoughts.

Nonetheless, God would not let me put the idea behind me. Each time I questioned Him, He pushed harder. Each time I tried to banish the thought from my mind, He placed it there with even more urgency. He would not allow me to let go of this. So, after much doubt and many questions, here is the story He has asked me to tell.

Suffice it to say that I am not capable of doing this on my own. It is only because of God that I am even capable of getting this many words on paper. If there is anything in this book that is good, it is because of the Lord. It is only through Him that this project has come to completion. God Himself has provided strength when I've needed it, and He has sent encouragement when I hit my lowest lows. Furthermore, He has placed people in my life to help me along the way—through their encouragement, proofreading, editing, praying, and believing that God will use this book to advance His kingdom.

I hope you enjoy this book—that you laugh and cry, reminisce and look ahead. I hope most of all that this story will reaffirm in your heart just how powerful God is. He is an awesome, wonderful God. I pray you will be blessed by this and that God will be glorified. He is an amazing God. To Him be the glory forever.

Contents

Chapter 1	Almost Time	11
Chapter 2	Pokeberries	18
Chapter 3	The Big Day	24
Chapter 4	Kowabunga!	32
Chapter 5	Recovery Room	38
Chapter 6	Day 2	45
Chapter 7	Leap of Faith	54
Chapter 8	Survival	61
Chapter 9	Day 3	70
Chapter 10	The Weather Bird	80
Chapter 11	A New Day	85
Chapter 12	Trampoline	95
Chapter 13	Home	99
Chapter 14	Trouble	106

Chapter 15	Checkup	112
Chapter 16	Learning to Drive	120
Chapter 17	Healing	126
Chapter 18	Four-Wheelin'	130
Chapter 19	Happy Birthday to Me	136
Chapter 20	Humbled	142
Chapter 21	No Fear	148

Chapter 1

Almost Time

It is two days before the big day. Part of me wants to surrender to the fear and let my emotions overtake me. I contemplate giving up on the tough fight and letting the panic and dread creep in and take control. I ponder the process that is going to take place soon. I cringe as I think about the pain that will follow and each challenge I will have to overcome. I know the path that awaits me will be filled with apprehension, anxiety, and fear.

Two days! So what do I do to take my mind off things? As I sit in our garage, I peruse the storage shelves looking for the answer to my question. I see my friend—an old, worn, leather basketball—sitting on a storage shelf. It has bounced on the ground so many times the leather is peeling and the words are fading. Most people would consider the ball trash, but I can't let go of it. Ironically, this old friend's betrayal is the source of my current anxiety. This nearly twenty-year friendship has taken a tremendous toll on my body. Not one to hold a grudge, I slap the worn leather against my palm, like a handshake.

I started playing basketball at age seven and retired at twenty-five, having played in grade school, high school, college, and professionally. Rarely did a day pass that I did not have a basketball in my hands. As a child I spent hours shooting in my driveway. I slipped on the wet asphalt when it rained and I shoveled when it snowed. That same driveway hosted hundreds of pickup games, many lasting long after darkness obscured our vision of the goal. In college we practiced at least once a day for sometimes more than three hours. We also had individual workouts with our coaches. Practice was very physical, as it was not uncommon to have a fellow teammate knock you to the ground or put a knee in your back during drills. Conditioning included weightlifting, running long distance, sprinting, and other activities to get our bodies prepared for the season.

Each day I put my body through much abuse. After college I played in the WNBA and overseas, including Finland,

Germany, Italy, and Hungary. The years of playing have damaged my back. Three of the discs in my lower back are herniated to different degrees. Also, the fluid in these discs has dissipated. At the age of twenty-four, the pain became so intense I realized I couldn't play much longer; my back would not let me. Shortly after that realization I sadly called it quits. I miss playing every day.

I take the basketball down off the shelf. I decide to see if I still "have it," and I'm all but sure I know the answer. I bounce the basketball between my legs and behind my back. It feels good, like old times. I keep going, reliving the old days when I played every day, all the time. God gave me both talent and a love for the game, and I enjoyed almost every minute. Of course there were bad days, but overall it was a wonderful, life-changing experience that will always be a big part of me. Those days were some of the best of my life.

Jack, my dog, has now become my defender. I use a crossover move on Jack and then put a step-back move on the four-wheeler. I hadn't touched a ball in over a year, and it's a good feeling until a sudden pain shoots down my left leg and stops me in my tracks. This intense pain, which so rarely vanishes, has changed my life. It makes me feel like my body is falling apart. It makes me feel like I can't go on. I want to throw in the towel and quit. As I fight through the pain and discouragement, I try to recall scriptures that will keep me going. "Therefore we do not lose heart. Though outwardly we are wasting away, yet inwardly we are being renewed day by day. For our light and momentary troubles are achieving for us an eternal glory that far outweighs them all" (2 Corinthians 4:16-17 NIV).

As I bounce the ball for just moments, I am reminded of why I haven't touched a basketball in a year. I am also reminded of what lies ahead for me. I will probably pay for the few minutes that I pounded that ball, but I don't care. In the morning I probably won't be able to get my socks on without help, but the few dribbles will be worth the pain. Two days from now I will not be able to do anything for awhile, so I should have a little fun while I still can.

In forty hours I will have back surgery, spinal fusion to be exact. Now don't get me wrong. I know things could be much worse. I know it could be something more serious, not to mention that this is supposed to make me better. I'm supposed to be able to dribble again. I'm supposed to be able to garden again and put my socks on without severe pain. I should be able to sprint for miles and miles and not have pain, not that I would. Sprinting ten feet is more than enough for me. Five a.m. meetings on the Western Kentucky University track in subfreezing temperatures have advanced my dislike for running. If you see me sprinting, a robber or a vicious dog will not be far behind.

I am scheduled to arrive at the hospital at 5:45 a.m. The hospital sits in the middle of town, a thirty-minute drive from my house. At 4 a.m. I will scratch and claw my way out of bed and compel myself to step into the shower. It will be a special shower for two reasons: it will be my last for a few days, and I am required to use antibacterial scrubbing brushes to prepare myself for the surgery. So I will scrub down, pack up, and head into town. When I step into our vehicle, I expect dread will be knocking at my mind's door. It knocks now, but I am trying to keep the door locked and intimidation out.

I struggle with not submitting to fear as I confront this obstacle in front of me. When I think about and talk about what the doctor will do, it is overwhelming. Just the mention of spinal surgery is intimidating, but when it is *your* spine, fear can overtake you. It was a few weeks before my surgery, and I was visiting Dr. Wood, my surgeon for my final appointment. The first time the surgery really "sank in" for me was when my doctor stretched out his fingers to show me the six-inch incision he would make. Sometimes, as the cliché goes, ignorance truly is bliss.

"So what exactly will you do to my back?" I asked.

Dr. Wood excused himself to go get a model of a spine. He reentered the room with a plastic spine in his hand. I glanced at the spine wide-eyed, thinking there were more rods and screws in it than you would see at a mechanic's shop. At least that's the way it looked when I imagined it being my own spine. Dr. Wood explained how he would drill holes in my vertebrae and then place the screws in the holes. He would then insert the rods through brackets in the screws. As I listened to him, my thoughts overwhelmed me. Ignorance was gone, replaced by the reality of what I would have to face.

I had ignored fear until that final doctor visit. Justin, my husband, and I had been busy traveling during the holidays, so I filled my thoughts with work and plans. I talked about the surgery, but I didn't admit to myself that it would actually take place. In my mind it was something so far away I didn't need to think about it. But now everything has changed. In about forty hours I will be lying on a cold table getting a CAT scan. I will cringe as the nurse starts the IV. I cringe now just thinking about it. IVs, in my opinion, are awful. My thoughts will start to run out of my control. Work and travel will not consume my thoughts as I change into my hospital gown and the people in masks and caps approach me.

Will everything go well? Will I be okay? Will I be able to handle the pain that will follow the surgery? Will I be able to live the active lifestyle I did before the pain got so bad? Will I be able to live without pain again? These are the questions I will entertain as I prepare for my surgery that day.

I do know this: my God knows the answers to all those questions as I write these words and wait for time to pass. "For I know the plans I have for you, declares the Lord, plans to prosper you and not to harm you, plans to give you hope and a future" (Jeremiah 29:11 NIV).

I know God will see me through this. I know He is with me. I believe in Him and in His power. I believe He casts out fear. Besides, I have never been the type to let fear direct my paths or influence my decisions. I am sure most of my family and friends would attest to that fact.

Chapter 2

Pokeberries

I was raised in a family that loves to eat. We celebrate everything with a meal. What else would you expect of folks from the South? We look for excuses to have a good meal. We have family dinners for most every holiday on the calendar, and we celebrate birthdays monthly with good food. My family is blessed with some of the best cooks known to man. We usually have all the fixin's when we eat together: mustard greens, corn, beans, and, if we're lucky, some homemade dumplins or noodles. We even have red-eye gravy on occasion. Depending on where you're from, you might or might not know what this is. "Red-eye" says it all since the gravy is made from coffee instead of milk, like traditional gravy.

All the wonderful meals my family made created in me a strong desire to cook some fabulous food of my own. I wanted to live up to the high standards of cooking that had been set in my family down through the generations. When I was around six years old, my friend and next-door neighbor, BJ, and I would pretend to indulge ourselves with mud pies. We would bake them to perfection and imagine eating the whole thing, then brag about what great bakers we were. We actually *did* eat them sometimes. I think the old saying "God made dirt, dirt won't hurt" applied to much of my childhood.

Since I liked making and eating these mud pies, I was always looking for new ingredients to make them even more wonderful. There were plenty of plants and vines to explore near our house. One day we found these small, delicate strawberries to put on our mud pies to top them off. I loved the strawberries I ate at home, so I knew these would be great. We completed our masterpiece with the petite, beautiful berries. When the mud pie was finished baking we would have our perfect dessert. We were both giddy because of the wonderful pie we had created as world-renowned bakers. We gave new meaning to "my little bakeshop."

If we found these strawberries, I guessed there were more toppings to be found. I was on the hunt again to find something new to delight my taste buds. I found a small, round, purple berry that grew around our storage building in the backyard. In my childish thinking, these would be ideal to use on our mud pies. These berries, I found out later, are commonly called "pokeberries."

I started eating the pokeberries. A taste test was vital before adding them to our mud pies. After BJ and I consumed a few, we started topping our pies with them. In our eyes it was perfection. I thought since we had made such a marvelous creation, we should show my mom. BJ agreed and we both ran toward my house filled with excitement over what we had done. We went in the back door and ran through the house until we found my mom.

"Mom, come and see our mud pies! They're wonderful," I said. "We found some berries down at the storage building to put on them."

At hearing these words a red flag went up for my mom. We weren't growing any berries, so she knew we had gotten into something that was not good. Mom didn't want to see our mud pies; she wanted to see what we were picking at the storage shed to put on them. She walked outside with us to

No Fear

see exactly what we had gotten ourselves into. We made our way down to the storage shed. When we got close Mom's face turned a bit pale.

"Have you been eating these?" she said, her voice filled with anxiety.

BJ and I just looked at each other. I'm sure Mom knew the answer to her question the second she saw our reaction. I could tell my mom was upset, but I wasn't sure what the big deal was. Shouldn't she be excited about our masterpiece pie? We were oblivious to the problem, but Mom understood, like most of the locals, that these beautiful berries were considered poisonous.

Mom turned and quickly made her way back into our house. BJ and I followed. My mom was clearly concerned. She rushed to the phone and called the poison control center. BJ and I sat at our kitchen table unsure and unsettled. We didn't understand what all the commotion was about. We were just baking mud pies.

"My daughter and her friend have eaten some berries growing outside our house," she said. "They are small, purple berries. I think they're called pokeberries."

There was a pause.

"No, I'm not sure how many," she said.

As I listened to my mom, I started to get worried, as the anxiety in her voice heightened. I wasn't sure what was going to happen, but I knew I had done something wrong. I heard her say "okay" a few times and then she hung up the phone. Mom looked at us, and I could see the worry in her face. BJ and I kept our eyes on her to see what was going to happen next.

Mom frantically dialed the phone again. Time was precious for everyone, and each turn of our rotary phone seemed to take forever. You could feel the tension radiating from my mom.

"I need you to go to the drugstore immediately and get some ipecac for me. I need it to induce vomiting for these kids who have eaten something they shouldn't have," she said to one of her good friends. "I need you to go right now."

My mom then called BJ's mom, Aimee, to tell her what had happened. Minutes later Aimee arrived, and we all waited. You could see the panic in our mothers' faces. As we waited for the antidote, seconds seemed like minutes and minutes like hours. Finally, my mom's friend came dashing in the door. We could not have been more relieved if the world's best doctor walked in.

BJ and I did not know it, but we were both in for a rough time ahead. The minute the ipecac made its way into our house, everything went downhill for us. Mom mixed our drink and we choked it down. I knew nothing good could come out of this and nothing did. The mixture was not pleasant, but what it did to you afterwards was even less pleasant.

After drinking the mixture, Aimee took BJ home. We became two sick little girls. Maybe the ipecac was a lifesaver, but my thoughts toward it did not include gratitude.

We had gone from a wonderful day of mud pies to a day of induced vomiting and sickness. I questioned the choice, of course, to tell Mom about our great mud pies as I puked my guts out. Now, though, as I look back on it, I realize it may have saved our lives. That choice led to the call to get instructions on how to clean our insides out. Alive and well, I soon would embark upon another wild adventure.

Chapter 3

The Big Day

The big day arrived. Morning broke and I went through my routine and headed out the door with Justin by my side. As we drove down the road I was especially observant. More observant than I'd ever been during this routine trip, because this day was anything but routine. It would be days or even weeks before I traveled this road again and enjoyed it. I knew this, and as a result I soaked up the scenery like a sponge. I saw the trees and hills, and their beauty spoke to me as never before. In each marvelous view I could see the hand of God. My eyes saw clearer than ever before the wonders He created.

When you believe there is even a miniscule chance you might not see tomorrow, you look at everything differently. I was thankful for views that might not have caught my attention before. I was thankful for the beauty God had placed before me, yet it is a tragedy that I had to face major surgery to appreciate such wonderful things I had taken for granted. I believed that my surgery would go well, but every alternate outcome ran through my head, over and over.

We arrived at the hospital at 5:45 a.m. Though I got out of the car, I fought the urge to run to the driver's side, push Justin out of the way, and drive as far away as I could. This impulse was hard to overcome as we crossed the parking lot. I was also tempted to do a little dance since I knew I wouldn't be able to move at all in a few hours. The urge overcame me, so I allowed myself one last dance before I entered the door. I tapped my foot a couple of times against the pavement and did a smooth sidestep. I don't even like to dance, but I could not resist the temptation. I just wanted to move a bit while I still could, and dancing seemed like a good outlet. I would have preferred throwing a ball or taking a swim, but that wasn't realistic in a hospital parking lot. I don't think anyone saw me, not even Justin, but if anyone did, he or she no doubt got a good laugh at my silly dance.

Upon entering the hospital, I went to the attendant's desk and gave her my name. She soon handed me an I.D. bracelet with my personal information and asked me to have a seat in the waiting area. Shortly thereafter a female technician in scrubs appeared calling my name. My time had come. My life would now change. As we walked back to the prep room, I felt like I was walking down a dark hallway toward a cold dungeon. A fifty-pound lump of dread formed in my stomach. My steps grew slower and slower as if concrete blocks encased my feet. I slogged on with Justin by my side. We finally arrived at my room, and I was handed a hospital gown and a plastic bag.

"Place all your clothes and belongings in this bag and wait here," she said.

"Can I leave my pants and socks on?" I asked. I knew I would be freezing in no time because of the cold hospital room and my increasing nervousness. The tech agreed and I changed into my gown and waited. Justin and I sat there quietly. The tech reentered a few minutes later with a cup and a pill.

"What's this?" I asked.

"Valium, to relax you before the surgery," she said, so I took it as instructed.

I struggled to control my thoughts and fears as we sat in the cold room. The last thing I needed was quiet time to think, but that is what I had. I lay there waiting, my mind running frantic with dreadful thoughts of pain and doubt that I wished would disappear. Would I make it through the surgery all right? Would I be able to endure the recovery? Would I be able to walk without pain again? Is this the right decision? All the questions that flooded my mind earlier rushed in like a tidal wave of anxiety. As I lay in the bed the door opened and my mom, grandpa, and Uncle Jerry arrived to be with Justin and me. I was relieved to see them. If nothing else, they would distract me. As they came in, I could see concern in their eyes, but I knew they were trying to disguise it with small talk and lighthearted teasing.

"Did you think this was the only way you could get a vacation?" asked my uncle, referring to my occupation in the family business.

For a moment the mood lightened. My spirits rose as I felt their genuine love for me. Moments later the joking ceased and everyone became quiet. I could feel the tension creeping in. The room became weighted down with anxiety.

Then my grandpa spoke up. "We can claim God's promises today." We all listened quietly as Grandpa reached inside his coat, brought out his Bible, and began to read. "Matthew 18:19-20 says, 'Again I say to you that if two of you agree on earth concerning anything that they ask, it will be done for them by My Father in heaven. For where two or three are gathered together in My name, I am there in the midst of them.' There are five of us gathered here today, and we agree that we want your surgery to go well, and we can claim that promise from God," he said. "I have prayed about this, and I believe that your surgery and recovery will go well and that you will be okay. We should thank God for His promises and that He is here today with us."

Tears filled my eyes as I listened to Grandpa say each word. After his words we all bowed our heads in prayer. Peace flooded my heart as Grandpa prayed. I listened as he thanked God for His promises to us. I rejoiced as he thanked God for what He was going to do for me. His words were sweet to my ears.

God had answered my prayers. I had asked Him on many occasions to grant me peace before the surgery and to take away my fears. He had done this, as His Word said He would. "And the peace of God, which surpasses all understanding, will guard your hearts and minds through Christ Jesus" (Philippians 4:7 NKJV). What a wonderful blessing to know that we can claim the promises of God and He will never fail us. I know that God was in the room that day, and I was reassured that He is with me everywhere.

Grandpa and Uncle Jerry left the room to stay with my little brother, Christian, so that my dad could come and see me. Christian, who was sixteen at the time, has cerebral palsy and needs someone to stay with him at all times. We are blessed to have a family who are there to help us whenever needed and in whatever way. Shortly after Grandpa and Jerry left, my dad arrived. His face held the same concern as the others' had. Their love and distress for me, coupled with my own apprehension, brought me again to tears. As I fought for composure, I recognized how blessed I am to have such a wonderful, loving family. I believed the procedure would go well, but knowing what lay ahead still brought on emotions and anxiety.

The technician returned, and I knew it was time for me to go. She maneuvered my bed around and wheeled it out the door as my family told me they would see me in a little while. I rolled down the hall to the operating room with a sense of peace. As they poked at me and hooked up the machines, I was able to joke with the nurses because of that peace. I relaxed as best I could, knowing what lay ahead.

"I'm going to get your IV started," the nurse said.

"Okay, if you have to," I said reluctantly.

The nurse started sticking my hand with the needle, but the IV did not go in easily. Earlier, at my request, the tech had placed a numbing agent on my hands so I would not feel the IV insertion, but unfortunately she had placed it in the wrong spot on my left hand. Consequently, I felt everything, and it was painful. After two tries on the left, the nurse switched to my right hand and had success. My right hand was numb in the correct spot, so it was not painful. I had survived my first of many challenges.

Nurses and other attendants moved all around me getting prepared for my surgery. Doors opened and closed, and equipment was pushed past me. Lines and cords were attached to my body, and machinery was put in its proper place. I could tell we were getting closer by the minute.

"You guys are going to need some sunglasses if you plan on being involved in my surgery," I told the nurses. "Many parts of my body are a blinding sight."

All the nurses and attendants who heard me laughed. I failed to mention that I was given the nickname "The Ghost" by some friends from college.

"We're going to give you something to relax," one nurse told me.

That would be the last thing I remembered of pre-surgery. It was time for a very long nap.

Chapter 4

Kowabunga!

The white house was my home growing up—a nice two-story house with a basement. You can guess why we called it "the white house." Oh, the adventures I had there. In my imaginary world, I could be Smokey from *Smokey and the Bandit* just by putting on my dad's brown "trucker vest," as I always called it. I could be Michael Jackson in "Thriller" with my diamond glove. With my vivid imagination, almost anything was possible at my house.

The white house sits in the small town of McKee, Kentucky. The population of McKee was roughly a thousand when I was growing up there, although I think it has increased now. I was blessed to grow up in a small town and enjoy the benefits of small-town life, such as fishing, pond swimming, and four-wheelin'.

The main floor of our house consisted of one bedroom, the living room, a kitchen, and a bathroom. The television sat in the living room, and I spent many hours engrossed in its fantasy worlds. I especially enjoyed cartoons, and one of my favorites was *Teenage Mutant Ninja Turtles*. If you remember this cartoon, then I have given my age away. *Teenage Mutant Ninja Turtles* was very popular in the late 1980s. Since lots of kids were watching it, and marketers were starting to realize the potential in children, you could buy Ninja Turtles Halloween costumes, video games, action figures, and plenty of other merchandise. I watched the turtles often, had their names memorized, and learned as much about each one as I could. Michelangelo was a cool character with a laid-back attitude, and he just happened to be my favorite turtle. Each turtle wore a bandana in his own unique color, and each had his own weapon. Michelangelo carried nunchakus and wore an orange bandana. He was by far the coolest of all the turtles.

As a kid I was always full of energy. Hyperactive is an understatement; I made the Energizer bunny look like a couch potato. My parents always tell me it was all they could do to keep up with me, but I sure kept them (and others) entertained. My entertaining did not always have good results though. There was never a dull moment when I was around. If I were quiet, it was time for my parents to investigate, for surely my silence meant that I didn't want them to know about something.

I can remember running through the white house spinning and kicking, defeating the bad guys in my imaginary world as Michelangelo the Teenage Mutant Ninja Turtle. I always won each fight. No bad guys could defeat Michelangelo, the best turtle of all. Until one day this "Michelangelo" met his match.

Michelangelo always yelled, "Kowabunga!" as he kicked and punched and destroyed his enemy, so therefore I did the same. I ran through our kitchen and yelled out, "Kowabunga!" as I kicked and punched the evil enemies that the turtles fought on TV. The fighting was intense, and I was in a hard battle. I was jumping and fighting with all my energy. As I moved around the kitchen I ran over to the glass storm door at the side of our house and yelled, "Kowabunga!" as I kicked the storm door. I was imagining Michelangelo's archenemy, but as I hit the door reality set in.

The enemy had overtaken me. I broke the glass in the door, but the glass also broke me. I cut my leg badly as it went through the glass and had numerous small cuts on my arms and hands. I was a mess. My mom heard the noise and came running. I was bleeding heavily and managed to scare my mother and her friend to death. Discussions about the emergency room and doctors went on between my parents and our guest. Mom wanted to take me to the emergency room, but Dad thought I would be all right. My mom's friend agreed to go with us to the emergency room. Mom started preparing to make the forty-five-minute trip. As she got us ready to leave, my bleeding slowed and Dad convinced my mom that I would be okay. I was cut badly, but my wounds would soon heal. Before long I was ready for my next fight, which, unfortunately for my family, occurred too soon. The storm door episode would not be the only time I would use my body as a battering ram against a glass door.

My family has been in the oil and gas business as long as I can remember. Our office sat in walking distance of the white house, with my grandparents' house in between. My mom worked and I stayed with my grandma on many days. The office had loading docks and a stockroom with cases of oil and other oil products. There was an abundance of things for me to climb and play on at our office.

The entrance to our office was a thick, solid glass door. At first sight you would believe it would take a sledgehammer to break through the door. It seemed almost indestructible, but the door hadn't run into me yet. I was playing on the loading dock one day, and all of a sudden, for no good reason, I ran toward the door. Even to this day I can't tell you exactly what my motivation was. I had again made a hasty decision without any thought. With all the energy I could muster I ran directly into the door. Glass went everywhere, and again I bled profusely. Our secretary, Cleva, was frightened when she heard the crash and saw me hit the door. I scared her so much that she was shaking uncontrollably.

After seeing me bleeding, Cleva asked for the remainder of the day off. Her husband took her home, as she was unable to work or drive because of the trauma I had caused her. I was cut up badly, but again I had no major injuries. I had numerous cuts and scratches, but the glass had missed all my major arteries and veins. I know God was watching over me. There is no other explanation for surviving everything I put my body through as a child.

I feel remorse for everything I put my mom through. There were so many times that she was overcome with fear and worry. She was there that day to slow the bleeding and bandage my wounds after my launch through the door. Life in the Lunsford household would have been much rosier if I had learned from my mistakes instead of repeated them.

Chapter 5

Recovery Room

"I need to pee," he said.

"Mr. Johnson, you have a catheter in. You can go ahead and pee," replied the nurse.

A short silence occurred.

"I need to pee," Mr. Johnson said again.

"Mr. Johnson, you have a catheter in. You can go ahead and pee," the nurse repeated.

"You're in the recovery room, Mrs. Mahoney," said my nurse.

The long sleep was over. It was 8:30 a.m. when they took me to pre-op, and I had made it—it was over. I pushed myself to regain a sense of reality. I couldn't quite grasp what was going on. I knew Mr. Johnson had to pee: that was clear to me. Or was it? Was this real or was I dreaming? Even though I was told I was in the recovery room, things seemed fuzzy. I guess anesthesia will do that to you. Mr. Johnson had to pee though, and he had made that evident at least five times. At this point I wanted to either walk over and reassure him that he had a catheter or show him the nearest restroom.

There wouldn't be any walking though, not now, only ice chips and morphine. The surgery was over and I was glad, but I knew I had a long road ahead of me. I dozed in and out of sleep, slipped in and out of reality.

A short time later my driver arrived to wheel me and my bed to my room. Down the halls we slowly went until we reached the elevator. I stared at the ceiling as we moved and became nauseated as I watched it flow by. We waited until the elevator arrived. When it did, we got on and headed for the fourth floor, my home for the next few days. We got off the elevator, and as we neared my room I saw my family; what a welcome sight! They stood at the end of the hallway waiting for me.

"I think she's out of it," I heard Justin say.

I raised my hand in a wave to tell him I was okay.

"I guess not," he said to my Uncle Jerry.

As we turned into my room, I saw my nannie sitting in the corner. These faces were a precious sight to my eyes. After I got settled in, numerous family and friends piled into my room. I can't explain the comfort I felt by seeing all their faces. Each face brought me a safe, familiar feeling. As I glanced around my temporary home, I saw a big clock on the wall: 4:30 p.m. Could it be? Had I really been unconscious that long? I was sure I hadn't been in pre-op or recovery for more than thirty minutes. I thought the clock must be wrong, otherwise it had been eight hours since they took me back for the surgery. I was sure it could not have been that long. I was wrong!

I could tell by my family members' expressions that I looked dreadful. I later asked my mom how I had looked. She said my face was very swollen and my eyes were kind of sunk back into my head. Since I had been lying on my stomach for several hours, this was normal. She also said that after she saw me, she felt sick and thought she would pass out. Seeing me that way was almost more than she could bear.

"What's wrong with your face?" asked my Uncle Jerry.

"I don't know," I replied.

I didn't know anything was wrong with my face, so I reached up to see if I could feel anything abnormal. I felt some watery bubbles on my forehead. Several blisters had appeared after my surgery, large enough that I could easily feel them. At the time I had no idea what had caused the blisters. Dr. Wood later told me I had thermometers taped to my face during the surgery. He guessed that I had an allergic reaction to the tape. My forehead was blistered, my eyes were glazed, and my mouth was parched.

I needed something to drink, but I was only allowed ice chips. I hate ice. I've got sensitive teeth and it hurts to have ice on them. In fact, often I order drinks without ice; however, after the surgery I couldn't get enough ice chips. Apparently anesthesia does that to me. My family and friends took turns feeding them to me. Justin stood over me and gently placed ice chips in the corner of my mouth. Then Mom took a turn and later on Dad did the same. The ice chips were the only thing I wanted, and I consumed them in mass quantities. I couldn't get enough of them since my mouth felt like I had eaten a plate of sand.

The nurses were working on my machines during this time, and the room was full of people. My grandpa approached me and asked if he could lead us in a prayer of thanksgiving. He said he would like to do that, but the room was busy with work. He indicated that he would wait until things slowed down a little bit before we prayed.

"Please do the prayer now, Grandpa," I said with what little strength I had.

I wanted everyone in the room—nurses, family, and friends—to be involved and hear Grandpa's prayer. The more the merrier. I thought we should all praise God's goodness together. I wanted everyone in there to know that we can claim God's promises and that He is with us always. This could have been the perfect opportunity for someone to hear about my God. I also wanted to thank God right away for what He had done for me. I didn't want to wait another minute. When you're being put to sleep, you have that concern about not waking up. I had awakened and I wanted God to know I was thankful for keeping me safe thus far.

As my grandpa prayed, I was overwhelmed with joy and thankfulness to a wonderful God in my life. I was humbled that He would even want to be in my life. As undeserving as I was, He still loved me. He was there for me and brought me through the surgery. We claimed God's promises that day that He would be with me and take care of me, and we thanked God for allowing us to claim them. Even if the surgery had not gone well I still knew that God would not leave me and that He would always take care of me.

Slowly, after prayer, the room thinned out until only Mom, Grandpa, and Nannie were left with me. Justin had gone to get some food since he knew I was doing all right. I lay flat on my back with a tube running out of my back to let fluid drain. I felt as though I were stuck in concrete. I could move my arms a little, but I could not move my legs or torso even an inch. I had expected limited mobility, but now I felt frustrated and helpless.

I wanted to tell Grandpa to thank people for praying for me, but when I looked at him I found myself unable to speak. I could not even get out one word. Instead, tears started to flow and I cried uncontrollably. I was consumed and overwhelmed by fear. My mom quickly came to the side of my bed.

"What's wrong?" she asked.

"I'm scared," I said.

"It will be okay," she said.

Grandpa stepped to the other side of my bed. "Remember we have claimed the promises of God. Everything will be okay. He is with you."

The stark realization of my immobility and vulnerability had set in and overwhelmed me with fear. Taking my mind off God and His Word for one moment had allowed fear to creep in. I truly believe we can trust God and claim His promises to us. I believe in His precious Word. I was very helpless now, but I was not alone. God has promised this to me. God was with me all along and would continue to be.

As Grandpa's comforting words penetrated my heart, I reset my focus and settled in for some much needed rest. This situation illustrates how easily we can be overtaken by fear. It also shows how powerful God is; by the mention of His Word I felt peace. "And let the peace of God rule in your hearts, to which also you were called in one body; and be thankful" (Colossians 3:15 NKJV).

Chapter 6

Day 2

"If you can survive the second day, then you will be okay," said my nurse.

When I first decided to do the surgery, I knew it would be tough. I dreaded it, but I didn't realize how difficult it was really going to be. When the nurse said "survive," she meant it. Not that I was literally close to death, but the days that lay ahead of me after the surgery would be very hard. I was incapable of caring for myself and severely weak. Day number two would be a challenge like I had never faced before.

The night after my surgery I slept very little. I strongly desired to sleep, but my discomfort made it an unattainable goal. I had the tube in my back, and the bed was comparable to a wood floor. After enduring a long, slow night the sun rose; I had made it to the second day.

The first face I saw that early morning was a technician, and she carried a needle. Have I mentioned how much I hate needles? I despise them. Just the thought of metal going into my skin and veins makes me a bit woozy. I could tell you story after story of me passing out after getting a routine flu shot or vaccine. I am a baby when it comes to needles. From the moment I decided to do the surgery, there have been needles. There were needles before the surgery, during the surgery, and now after the surgery. I came to my senses that morning just in time to see the tech coming toward me with her needle. With every step she took my heart sank. She repeated this ritual every single morning. By the third day I questioned whether I could refuse this morning routine. I learned I could, but I decided to try to endure it, knowing there had to be a good reason for it. The last two mornings, my eyes filled with tears each time the tech walked in the door. I hate needles!

After straightening my arm, inserting the needle, and drawing my blood the technician disappeared out the door. At this point in my recovery journey, I was unable to roll, turn, or do anything by myself. I had to wake Justin numerous times, asking him to roll me or move me just a little. It was almost unbearable lying on my back for so many hours. The tube in my back also increased the discomfort and immobility. I was very careful to keep the tube hidden under my sheets and tried to never look at the drainage seeping through it. Keep in mind: this is the girl who passed out after cutting her finger. This is the girl who passed out after getting her ears pierced as a teenager. After the piercing at a jewelry store, I walked over to look at the watches. I bent over the glass case for a closer look, feeling a little lightheaded. In the process I passed out. No one around me came to my rescue because they thought I was just taking a really close look at the watches. Knowing this, who could expect me to appreciate the blood-and-fluid-filled tube or the morning visits from the technician?

Dr. Wood came in to tell me how the surgery went.

"How are you doing?" he asked.

"I'm okay," I said.

"Your surgery went well. You did good during the surgery. We only had one small problem, but I don't expect it to cause any difficulties. One of the screws that we put in your spine was off about a millimeter, but I checked and it's not hitting any of the nerves. You would not know it if I hadn't told you, but I really don't think it will cause you any future problems."

"How big are the screws?" Justin asked.

Dr. Wood started feeling around in his pocket.

"I thought I might have a pencil, but I don't. The screws are about the size of a No. 2 pencil," he said.

"That's bigger than I expected," Justin said.

Dr. Wood asked if we needed anything else and answered a few minor questions for us, then he was on his way to his next patient.

My next visitor was a nurse that I hadn't remembered ever being in my room before.

"I'm going to take your catheter out," she said as she walked to the side of my bed.

I nodded agreeably. I knew this meant I would have to get out of the bed soon, and I did not look forward to that. I assumed this action took place so that I would have to get up and get moving a little. I had always heard that they try to get you going as soon as possible. I'm sure it's a positive thing to get you moving, eating, and trying to get back to a somewhat normal life. At this point I wasn't moving or eating, but things were about to change.

On the day of the surgery I was allowed no food or liquid, but now the ban had been lifted. I desired food as much as I desired seeing the tech and her needle come through the door. My appetite was nonexistent, and for me that is unusual. There are not many times that I don't want to eat, or can't eat, but this was one of them. All I really wanted was a Coke to ease my parched mouth. Although my appetite was gone, my family's desire for me to eat was stronger than ever. Luckily, my breakfast got misplaced and food did not arrive until lunchtime.

My mom, Nannie, Grandpa, and Uncle Jerry came to see how I was doing. Their faces were again a welcomed sight. They arrived just in time to join Justin in trying to get me to eat the turkey sandwich that had been delivered to my room.

"You have to eat something," Justin said firmly.

"You need to build up your strength," my nannie persuaded.

This entourage continued to coerce me, so I finally gave in. Since I could not feed myself, Justin fed me small bites of the turkey sandwich. I choked down as much as I could until my stomach could not take anymore.

Family and friends were in and out all day. I needed their support, encouragement, and presence. What a blessing from the Lord to see their beautiful, smiling faces and to hear their uplifting words! I believe God used them to help me overcome the fear I had. Likewise, when I awoke at night, the sight of Justin in the chair beside me comforted me. What a great blessing from God!

My parents, grandparents, brother, and uncle planned to return home on this day. I had encouraged them to leave, as I knew they had been through a lot also. I was sure they were tired, as they were spending their nights in a hotel and needed to go home to get some rest. Also, my brother is always ready to get home. It is his favorite place, where he is the most comfortable. After some reassurance from me that I was okay, they left and went to the hotel to pack. Justin and I were alone when the physical therapist arrived after lunch.

"We need to get you up and walking," he said as he walked into the room.

"I don't think I can do it," I said.

Looking as if he had heard that before, he said, "Yes, you can. We need to get you up and moving."

I was sure I wasn't ready for "up and moving," but who was I to argue? I didn't have the energy or strength to argue.

I concluded it was best just to get it over with. I lay there as the therapist prepared the room for my first walk. After everything was out of the way, Justin and the therapist raised me from my back to a sitting position on the side of the bed. I knew immediately that "up and moving" was not a good idea. I felt overwhelmed with dizziness and weakness, and I was sure I would fall over onto the floor even before I got up.

"I can't do this," I said.

"It will be okay. We won't go far. We'll just have you walk around to the other side of the bed to the chair," he said.

This guy was persistent.

"I can't do this," I said.

So was I.

"Yes you can. Let's just go to the chair," he pressed.

I was sure at this point that the guy wasn't going to relent. I was also sure I couldn't put up much of a fight. At six-foot-two I am a big girl, and a couple of days ago I could have taken him, but now there was no chance. I reluctantly complied. As soon as I sat up on the side of the bed, I felt sure I would pass out. I was too weak, but nobody would listen. I devised a plan in my head. I would attempt to get up, and once on my feet I would shoot for the world's record for fastest walk around a hospital bed after major surgery. If I didn't, I knew I would end up on the floor, and I did not want that. One surgery was enough for me this week.

As I rose to my feet with help from the PT and Justin, I knew it was coming. With Justin on one side of me and the physical therapist on the other, I walked as fast as I could. In my mind I looked like one of those speed walkers with their legs pumping and their arms swinging back and forth, but in reality I think I looked like a cross between a dog just hit by a car and a baby learning to walk. I don't know if I broke the record, but I do know I arrived just in time. I fell into the chair.

"I'm going to pass out," I said.

"It's okay. You're in a chair," said the physical therapist.

His words failed to comfort me. I didn't want to pass out even if I was in a chair. And then, I was out! I am not sure how long I was out, but I don't think it was very long. When I regained consciousness, several people were standing over me. Then I saw Justin. In our ten years of marriage, I had never seen him look so pale and worried. When I saw his face it scared me. He looked like he had seen a ghost. I could hear everyone talking, but I couldn't digest what any of them were saying. The nurse took my blood pressure and immediately called the doctor while I tried to recover.

"Please put me back in the bed," I pleaded. "I need to lie down."

"Just a few minutes," Justin said.

"Please put me in the bed," I begged.

"Just a minute," Justin said. "The nurse will be back soon."

The nurse reached Dr. Wood, and he told her to administer Narcan, a drug that's used for cleansing the body of anesthesia and other medicines. He thought the drugs caused my drop in blood pressure and subsequent fainting. My blood pressure had plummeted to 72/31 and my heart rate was 45 bpm after my fainting spell. At the time, I didn't care what they gave me; he could have given me anything and I would not have cared. I just wanted to get back in the bed. I didn't have the energy to hold myself up in the chair, and though I wasn't even sure I could make it to the bed, I definitely wanted to try. Justin and the nurse finally helped me to the bed. After the nurse administered the Narcan, all was calm for the moment, but I didn't realize what effects this medicine would have later that night.

Chapter 7

Leap of Faith

Growing up in a small town, I lived differently than most. Standard social and recreational activities included fish fries, four-wheelin', and week long revivals. But when I mention these activities or pastimes to urban dwellers, they often look at me as if I'm speaking a foreign language. I had ample opportunities to enjoy these and various other rural "cultural" activities that are privileges to being a "country girl," including regular church attendance.

Like many of my childhood friends, I grew up in the church. For as long as I can remember I've been going to church. I have fond memories of my hometown church, McKee Baptist. I have been blessed and enriched by the wonderful people of this church. As I awaited my surgery,

I longed to have my small-town church family walking through this tough time with me. In the past, whenever my family has experienced illness and hardship, we've always had friends from church right beside us to offer support and a shoulder to lean on. I'm so thankful for what each and every one has done for my family. I currently attend a large church, and I have found it to be much harder to develop those close relationships when there are so many members. Yes, there are problems and disadvantages in small-town churches, as with anything else, but in my opinion the advantages clearly outweigh the negative aspects.

Our church sat one block off the main strip in town. Numerous steps led up to the front door, and upon entering, the pastor's office was to the right and an open doorway to the left. The doorway on the left could either take you to the basement or to the balcony. If you walked forward after entering the church you would pass through a large double doorway into the sanctuary. At the front, past rows of oak pews with green upholstery, stood the podium. Directly behind it were the choir pews. To the right of the podium sat the piano on which my mom played many songs. To the left sat the organ on which Dottie, the church's organist, made her music.

If you asked Dottie about me, she would tell you that her shoes always disappeared when I was around. When she played the organ, she preferred to remove her shoes so that her feet touched the organ pedals. The door I used to go from Sunday school to the sanctuary was beside the organ, so if her shoes were there when I was coming out from class I would snatch them and move them to a pew or take them with me. Because of this, she would have to walk to her pew barefoot after worship. She was kindhearted and took it well. I thought it was funny, but I'm not sure what some church members thought as she strolled through the church with no shoes on. If someone had visited from the city, they might have believed the vicious rumor about mountain people not wearing shoes. I'm glad she had a forgiving, pleasant attitude about it.

In addition to playing piano for the church choir, Mom had a trio with two of her friends. The choir usually practiced an hour or two before the Sunday night service. I would go with my mom to these practices. While Mom made beautiful music, I ran around and played. My friend Candi, whom I had known all my life, usually came with her mom, Peggy, who sang in the choir and the trio. During these rehearsals, Candi and I played throughout the church.

I was a rambunctious and mischievous child, which may be obvious by now. I constantly sought out exciting ways to expend my excess energy. It was a rare occasion for me to get tired. For me, a "timeout" was complete torture. I wanted to go, go, and go some more.

While our moms were busy rehearsing, Candi and I found many adventures. Actually I found the adventures, and Candi conspired with me. A lot of the action occurred in the balcony. During choir practice, Candi and I had it all to ourselves, which suited me perfectly.

Back in the foyer, after you entered through the doorway giving you the choice of balcony or basement, you could go left and head up two sets of stairs into the balcony. After the first set of stairs there was a big platform that the steps wrapped around as they went up. It was always fun to climb and play on that platform. We would go to the balcony, climb over on the platform, and jump off the other side. This was so much fun that we could entertain ourselves for long periods of time.

At the top of the steps the balcony opened up. There were always chairs and stage extensions in the balcony. As you reached the top, you could see everything going on down below in the sanctuary. It was probably ten or twelve feet from the top to the floor below. If you bent down low enough, no one could see you when you entered the balcony, as there was a wall around three feet tall at the front of the balcony for safety. I think the fact that no one could see us drew me to the balcony. Maybe my mom couldn't see me, but she knew when I was up there, and I would bet Candi's mom knew she was there too.

I always wanted to go to any practice with my mom. This meant plenty of time to spend with friends and play. This also meant some anxiety for my mom. Though she needed to concentrate, her mind was probably always on me. I'm sure she constantly wondered what I was into and exactly where I was. Our church was not large at all, but there were plenty of places to run and play. How much trouble could a kid get into at church anyway?

On occasion I had looked up at the balcony and wondered what it would feel like to jump off the top of it. While I really wanted to do it, I knew I must keep my plan a secret. I would have to achieve perfect timing and be aware of adults in the area. I would have to consider which adults were there as I prepared to put my plan into action. If any adult saw me or knew of my scheme, they would surely try to stop me. I pondered all this as I waited for the perfect time to arrive.

I cannot imagine what Candi's thoughts were as I revealed my plan to her. We approached the balcony and I said, "We need to stay low so that no one can see us."

At this point she ducked to a crawl, and so did I. I crawled over to the middle of the balcony right above where the big church clock sits and quickly climbed onto the wooden banister. Candi watched me make my way to the top. I also wonder what thoughts filled the choir members' minds as they looked up and saw a child on the banister. As soon as I got in position I was over the edge and down to the floor. I was Superman, if only for a moment, until I landed. I smacked the floor, and I knew instantly that the smack of discipline would soon follow. I was aware that I must quickly make my way anywhere other than that sanctuary.

"Daricia Shea!" I heard after I hit the floor hard and rolled into a ball. My mom had called my first name, which was never good. From there everything went by so fast. I rolled backwards toward the doorway leading to the balcony or basement and made a quick exit to the basement. I knew I needed to find a secure hiding place. I had jumped off the balcony during choir practice, so my mom had a decision of whether to remain in choir practice or find me and discipline me. I hoped she would choose the choir practice, but if not I prayed she wouldn't be able to find me. I didn't consider it at the time, but I was just delaying the inevitable. Since my dad was at home, which I made sure of before I jumped, I didn't have to fear him at the moment.

For the choir members who saw me jump, I'm sure their hearts sank. To look up and see a child flying off the balcony had to be scary. I'm sure they were filled with fear until they realized it was me. I can hear them saying, "It's just Shea again." Choir practice was interrupted so my mom could make sure I was not hurt. She found me, as parents always do, and made sure I was okay. After seeing that I was well and giving me a look that only a mother can, she returned hastily to choir practice.

My mom didn't see me jump, as she was reading her music and playing the piano at the time, but she would tell me later that the minute she heard the WHOP! on the floor, she knew it was me. I guess it was a mother's intuition, or it could have been that I was the only kid in the church crazy enough to do such a stunt. She wasn't too worried since she had grown accustomed to my senseless actions. Everyone else in the sanctuary may have suspected me too. I had managed to disrupt choir practice as never before. The story of the wild child who jumped off the balcony would live on for years.

Chapter 8

Survival

It was a remarkable achievement for me to make it back to my bed. I made it, but I needed all the help I could get. I lay there resting and watching the color come back into Justin's face. I was so relieved to just lie down in the bed. Weak and exhausted, I felt as if I had just run a marathon.

The remainder of the early afternoon was uneventful, which I greatly appreciated. My family returned from packing their belongings to find me worse than when they had left. As a result, their eagerness to return home changed to worry and a reluctance to leave. I knew I would have to be very persuasive to get them to go home. I told them time after time that I would be okay. The worried expressions on their faces let me know that the way I looked did not agree with the words I said. After a long debate I finally convinced them, insisting numerous times that I would be fine.

A severe thunderstorm, with the possibility of tornados, was due to arrive the next day, and I didn't want them to be in a hotel or traveling when it hit. They reluctantly agreed, but first they went shopping to get me some snacks from the grocery store, hoping I would eat them. The game of trying to get me to eat was played out each day I was in the hospital. Mom dropped off the snacks while Dad stayed with Christian in the van. Then Mom left to stay with Christian while Dad visited me once more before they left. Once my blood pressure returned to normal, I was able to rest most of the afternoon.

My rest was short-lived however, as another challenge loomed. I saw it coming, but I was powerless to stop it: I had to use the bathroom. I had held it as long as I could, not wanting to get out of bed. I had purposely drunk very little so I could stay in bed as long as possible. I had some Coke to try and ease the dryness in my mouth, but I didn't drink much. As the pressure on my bladder increased, I knew I was going to have to face this, so I asked Justin to get my nurse. He left and the two of them shortly returned.

"How do you want to do this?" she asked me.

I knew my choices were few, and my mind churned to try and devise the best plan with the least movement.

"I don't think I can make it to the bathroom," I said.

"Do you want me to put a bedpan under your hips?"

"I know I can't raise up at all," I said. "I think that would cause me severe pain even if you raised my hips for me."

I also knew I would end up with a wet bed, which would mean a change of bed sheets and me having to get totally out of the bed for more than a few seconds—something I could not endure.

"What about a potty-chair?" she suggested.

"I'll try, but I'm not sure I can even make it to a potty-chair," I said.

"I'll get one and we'll see."

My nurse left the room and returned with a potty chair. This would be my first potty-chair experience, and as she brought it in the door I could not believe I was in this situation. I couldn't believe I was this weak, this dependent, and this immobile. Justin and my nurse slowly raised me up. Every move hurt badly, and as soon as I was raised from a reclined position I got very dizzy. Unable to move any further, I sat on the side of the bed feeling woozy and nauseated.

"Can you make it to the chair?" Justin asked.

"I don't think so," I said.

I knew that standing would put me back to the ground quickly, as I would pass out again. Unable to stand, I grudgingly asked the nurse to hold a bedpan for me. I must say this was humiliating. I could not go any farther than the bed. Justin held onto me and I slid to the side and let my body hang off just enough to reach the pan. This was by far one of the most embarrassing moments in my life. I regretted letting them remove my catheter. Here I was on the side of the bed with my nurse, whom I had only met less than twenty-four hours ago, holding a bedpan for me. I was so thankful for the wonderful, loving care that each nurse gave me. They gave their all and helped me with every tough obstacle I faced. As I sat there, I was learning humility in a way I never would have imagined.

Justin and my nurse carefully slid me back into the bed. I was exhausted and embarrassed. I apologized to my nurse as she finished up in my room and headed for the door. I knew this was her job, but I felt like a burden to her. I lay there in my hospital bed wondering if I could make it through all this. I lay there unable to see any light at the end of the tunnel.

My nurse returned soon after and informed us that Dr. Wood suggested a blood transfusion. Apparently I had lost a lot of blood during the surgery and my body needed replenishment. This was part of the reason for the dizziness, lightheadedness, and weakness. *If I need a blood transfusion, why are they taking my blood every morning?* I thought. I have to admit her words scared me. Neither Justin nor I welcomed the idea of someone else's blood filling my body. In the state I was in, I was not capable of making major decisions. Justin would have to step in for me, and I trusted him with this decision, knowing he would educate himself and make a wise choice. He decided against the transfusion, which I was fine with, thus we waited for my body to replenish itself.

As afternoon faded into evening, my rest turned to restlessness. Around 7 p.m., Justin went to our house to get some clothing and feed our dogs, Buddy and Jack. My friend Belle had offered to stay with me during Justin's absence. I was starting to feel some discomfort in my back and legs when he left, but it was bearable. However, by 8 p.m. the pain had intensified substantially, and I was not sure I could endure it much longer. At this point I could hardly move my upper body other than my arms. I could move my legs a little now, so I bent them one after the other trying to find some comfort. I knew I could not stand much more of this. I was in misery. Clearly, the medicine used to remove the anesthesia and painkillers had done a superb job. I was writhing in pain, moving my legs and arms in an effort to cope.

"We've got to get you some help," Belle said.

"Press the call button and get a nurse," I said. "I need help now! I can't stand this anymore."

Belle pushed the call button numerous times to no avail. No one answered. No nurse appeared. No help arrived. We would find out later the call button was broken. After what seemed like an eternity, Belle left the room to track down a nurse herself. She left and returned quickly with news that she found a nurse and asked her to find my own nurse. A few minutes later my nurse appeared.

"What's wrong?" she said.

"Her pain has gotten so bad she can't stand it anymore," Belle said.

"I can't give her anything without orders from her doctor," said the nurse. "I'll page him immediately."

My nurse left the room, and Belle tried rubbing my legs to ease the pain. She persevered as thirty minutes elapsed and the nurse reappeared saying she had not heard back from Dr. Wood. It was about 9 p.m. at this point, and I didn't know how much longer I could endure the pain. I was overwhelmed mentally and physically, yet I had no choice but to stay the course. I was so distraught from the pain that I could not think clearly. I silently pleaded to God for help to persist and for the pain to subside.

"Please get me some help," I said repeatedly to Belle.

"They're trying to contact the doctor, sweetie," she said. "Hopefully he'll call back soon."

I was completely exhausted. I had a terrible fear that the pain would not get better or go away. I feared I had made a terrible choice in doing the surgery. I feared that I wouldn't get through it all. Not only was my battle physical, it was also mental. How could I go on like this?

Justin reappeared and Belle updated him on my situation. He and Belle rubbed my legs to ease the pain. Looking back, I think that is what helped me get through the intense pain. The pain was worst in my legs, and that little bit of relief helped more than they could know.

At 10 p.m. Belle had to leave. Justin continued to rub my legs to relieve some of the pain. My nurse checked on me periodically and updated me on her progress or, in this case, her lack of progress. She was doing all she could, but she still had heard nothing from Dr. Wood.

Around 11:30 p.m. the nurse came back in.

"Dr. Wood just called," she said. "He has approved a morphine pump for you. I'll get your pump going as soon as possible."

It was around midnight before my nurse was able to get the morphine pump going. When the pain started to ease I was filled with relief and then total exhaustion. I had survived, but looking back I'm not so sure how. For almost four hours I suffered intense pain. Seconds turned into minutes and minutes into hours. I had been in pain worse than this in my life, but never for such a long period of time. The pain mentally and physically broke me down. I didn't know how I was going to get through the distress. I didn't know if I could survive.

I did make it to the next day, but I was battered. I had been through so much that day. God once again saw me through and gave me relief when I felt like I could not go on. I was broken and thankful. "And not only that, but we also glory in tribulations, knowing that tribulation produces perseverance, and perseverance, character, and character, hope. Now hope does not disappoint, because the love of God has been poured out in our hearts by the Holy Spirit who was given to us" (Romans 5:3-5 NKJV). He calmed the fears that swirled through my mind and overwhelmed me with His peace. He brought me through. He reminded me that He is always with me, even when times are hard. He never leaves us, and He never left me. Thank You, Lord!

Chapter 9

Day 3

I had survived the second day after my surgery. My nurse assured me that if I could do that, things would start looking up. I thought now that I would begin to see the light at the end of the tunnel. As that light began to show, guess what I saw? That's right. It was 4:30 a.m. and the tech with the needle was headed for my vein. I wanted to tell her, "No, you can't have my blood today. I need my blood." I wanted to ask her never to come back again. I wanted to run, but I couldn't even get out of the bed on my own. I chose restraint and said nothing to the tech; I was just trying to get the process over with. She completed her job and quietly headed out the door. I tried again to get some rest.

Dr. Wood entered my room later that morning to check on me and talk with Justin and me. He wanted to discuss the option of getting a blood transfusion.

"I really want you to reconsider having the blood transfusion," he said. "This is something that can really help you to feel better faster and help you to heal."

"Won't her body make the blood it needs on its own?" Justin said.

"It will, but it can take a lot more time. The transfusion will help you feel better immediately," Dr. Wood said.

"We're concerned about problems that might occur from having the transfusion," Justin said.

"The chances of contracting a disease such as AIDS are one in a million. The blood is tested multiple times and is very safe," Dr. Wood said. "Because she lost so much blood, her body really needs help in recovering."

Dr. Wood answered all our questions and calmed the fears we had about the transfusion. He encouraged us to reconsider the decision, and we did—the benefits far outweighed the risks.

Around 11 a.m. my lunch arrived. I had no appetite so I did not look forward to the arrival of any meal. Meals had become bargaining events between Justin and me.

"You'll get out of here sooner if you eat more," he would say.

As much as I wanted to get home, I just couldn't eat much. I did not want anything to eat. It was not fun to try to eat when my body had no desire for it. After my light lunch, it was time for physical therapy again.

I did not have the same therapist as I had the day before. I wondered if my first therapist read my mind and sent someone new. After my first therapy session I had asked Justin to protect me if the first PT came back. I wanted Justin to tell him I wasn't getting out of bed and walking unless I was ready. I even wanted Justin to guard me if the PT was as persistent as he had been earlier. Justin is a big guy, so I knew I would be protected when the PT returned. In order for Justin to agree with my proposal, I had to promise one thing. He made me guarantee that I would give a 100 percent effort for physical therapy. He just wanted me to try since he knew I needed to start walking. I was fine with walking; I just didn't want to pass out again. Our pact was completed.

"Today we are going to see if you can use the walker and go down the hall a short way," my physical therapist said.

"Are you sure about this?" I asked, recalling the previous day's physical therapy session, which ended abruptly with my fainting.

"We'll catch you if you fall. I'll have a belt around your waist to keep you upright," she said.

Her words were not reassuring. My physical therapist was probably five-foot-five and I am six-foot-two. I looked at her trying to imagine her holding my tall frame drooping over a belt. I couldn't, but I knew Justin would be close, and he could hold me up.

Justin and the PT helped me to a sitting position. Dizziness soon followed. My PT placed a wide belt around my waist. I rose slowly to my feet with help from Justin, my therapist, and my hospital bed. Was it possible to be so weak and helpless? The walker was placed in front of me and it was time to go. I quickly became lightheaded, but with the speed of a tortoise I dragged my foot for the first step. I had made my pact with Justin, and I didn't want to disappoint him. I was sure I knew how babies feel when they are learning to walk; I just hoped I didn't topple like they do.

"Are you okay?" my PT asked.

"I think so," I said.

I still felt somewhat lightheaded, but less so than the day before. It was very scary to get out of bed, knowing the last time I had collapsed into a recliner. I thought staying in the bed sounded much better, but the medical staff didn't agree with me.

I took baby steps and made it to the door. A whole new world awaited me. I had spent forty-eight hours staring at the same walls, so a hallway never looked so good. I had no idea what lay outside my door. It was exciting to look at something new — even if that "something" was a hospital hallway. My standards for excitement were quite low. I could barely walk, so to make it out the doorway was an extreme challenge that I had overcome.

We started down the hall to the big glass windows at the end. My room was near the end, so they were not far. I was trying to reach those windows so I could see the outside world again. Though I had a window in my room, the closest I had been to it was my collapse into the recliner. I could see the clouds from my bed, but not much else. How wonderful it would be to lay my eyes on trees and grass. With each step I inched closer to the big windows. Justin was on one side and the PT on the other. When I reached them, what a wonderful sight to behold! The view was both pleasant to my eyes and uplifting to my soul. The bare trees and cloudy skies filled me with hope that I would regain my place in the outside world. I could almost smell the fresh air as I gazed out the large window. I was ecstatic to have made it this far. This same view would have meant nothing to me a couple of days ago, but now it was marvelous. "Holy, holy, holy is the Lord Almighty; the whole earth is full of his glory" (Isaiah 6:3 NIV).

After a few moments of gazing I turned and started back to my room.

"How are you doing?" said my physical therapist.

"Good except for the pain in my legs."

"How bad is the pain?"

"It's bad, but it gets worse with every step I take," I said.

"Let's get back to your room, and I'll let the nurses know so they can tell Dr. Wood," she said.

I returned to my hospital room with both a sense of hope and a feeling of complete exhaustion. The PT unhooked the belt and helped me back into bed. I'm not sure a bed could have felt any better. Yes, even a hospital bed. I was relieved to finally lie back down. After my workout, I just wanted to rest.

My nurse came in later to say that Dr. Wood was concerned about blood clots because of my leg pain. He ordered an ultrasound on my legs to rule out any clots. She also inquired about my bathroom usage or lack thereof.

"You need to get some fiber and laxatives if you haven't had a bowel movement before you go home," she said.

When I heard the words "fiber" and "laxative," I zoned out. Had she really just said that? I was thirty-one, not eighty-one. Fiber and laxatives are what I see at my grandparents' house. Could she really be serious that I might need those? Want something to make you feel older? Let someone talk to you about fiber or laxatives. I looked over and Justin was taking notes, so I decided to remain zoned out of this conversation.

"I'll be back with your blood in just a minute," my nurse said as she walked out.

I lay still and relaxed to let my body regain some of its strength. Phones rang occasionally and visitors appeared, but things were quiet. My nurse reappeared shortly with a unit of blood for me. A special thanks to anyone who has ever given blood. After a few minutes she got my transfusion started.

"You should start feeling better real soon," she said.

Those were welcome words, as a trip to the potty-chair currently felt like a triathlon to me: sitting up in bed was the cycling leg, standing up and moving to the chair was the swim, and the final exhausting leg to rise back up and sink gloriously into my bed was like the road race.

After receiving two units of blood, I could tell a difference. I felt somewhat less fatigued and weak. Good thing, because it was time for a trip to the basement for the ultrasound and X-ray. My driver arrived, unlocked the wheels on my bed, and rolled me out the door with Justin following. It was good to be out of that room, even if just for a trip to the basement.

We exited the elevator and made our way to the destination. Geez, it was frigid down there. A man met me and guided my bed into the X-ray room as Justin waited outside. I began to shiver as we entered the room.

"Do you want some extra blankets?" a woman inside the room said.

"Yes," I chattered.

"Can you crawl over to this X-ray table?" the man asked.

Was he serious? Did he really just say that? I could barely get out of bed with the help of two people.

"No, I can't," I said.

"Okay, we'll just pick you up with the sheets and move you over to the table."

They carefully placed me on the X-ray table. After the X-ray he did an ultrasound on my legs and moved me back to my bed. He then rolled me out the door to meet my driver and Justin. We made our way back through the halls.

"I bet you don't want to go that way," my driver said as he nodded toward a couple of doors. "That's surgery."

"No," I said. "Get me far away from there."

After a short elevator ride and a few steps down the hall, I was wheeled back into my room. I just wanted to rest, and rest I did. After a few hours I asked Justin for a pen and paper. I needed to write down what I was feeling at this moment. I wanted to capture my thoughts and emotions. I wrote:

The power of God is revealed to us as we become helpless. I have slowly watched myself go from a powerful, tough individual to a person who is trying to learn to walk again. That's when you know you're not in control, in control of anything. I think sometimes when things are going well and we are on top of the world, we get a false sense of security. We have a feeling that we can control things. And sitting on the hospital bed preparing to take my first steps let me know that, among other things, I was and am broken, and God and God only is in control. Praise the Lord that a God who loves us is in control.

I lie in my hospital bed and weep. Weep, because of the love of the Lord, because of the love of the Lord through others. I am blessed beyond measure. Physically, I have never been more broken than now. I have a long road ahead of me, but as I become more and more broken, I feel the power of my great God more. I see Him in my family. I see Him in gifts given to me. How wonderful He is, and how wonderfully He has provided.

It's amazing how God can use situations and circumstances. We spent the remainder of the night visiting friends and watching a little TV. I slowly dozed off to sleep, and dreams filled my head. I wanted to dream about flowers and puppies, but instead my thoughts were filled with the woman who awakened me each morning with her needle, which seemed to grow larger each day.

Chapter 10

The Weather Bird

My cousin Steph and I spent a lot of time together when we were kids. We had to have everything the same—toys, clothes, and all other gifts. If I got something and she didn't, she would cry and scream like a baby. I did my fair share of crying, screaming, and acting like a baby too when she received something that I did not. Our birthdays are close, so many times we got the exact same gifts. We would put our birthday gifts to good use and play for hours with our matching toys. This was a blessing to our family; with something to entertain us, we would stay out of trouble.

As kids, we did find time to get into some mischief. We often could be found jumping on the beds or the couch. We would throw all the cushions off the couch and build a fort with them. We talked Steph's brother, Jerome, into giving us rides on his back. He would get on all fours, and we'd climb on and hang on as tightly as we could. This did not create trouble until I decided to take a chunk out of his back with my teeth. He didn't appreciate this very much and sent me flying into the china cabinet. Steph and I were known for biting from time to time.

This day, like many others, was a day when our whole family was gathered at my grandparents' house for a family meal. My grandparents' house was a two-story with a basement that was used for canning vegetables and for storage. The upstairs had a couple of bedrooms and was one of our favorite places to play when at Nannie and Grandpa's. That's because it was away from the adults, who usually congregated downstairs on the main floor.

My Aunt Trish had bought a weather bird that resided upstairs. A weather bird is a glass-blown bird filled with liquid that changes colors to give you a weather report. For instance, the liquid inside the bird would turn blue if it was going to rain, or it would turn yellow for sunny weather. It was like having your own weatherman at home. I thought this bird was truly the coolest.

One day when all of our family was gathered, I decided Steph and I should conduct an experiment. We were upstairs playing and I got the weather bird from its resting place. I shook it to see what it would do. I turned it upside down to watch for a change in colors.

"Let's drink it," I suggested. I had already made up my mind what I was going to do, regardless of Steph's reply.

"Do you think we should?" she asked.

"Yeah, it will be okay," I said.

I did not wait for her compliance. I broke the neck on the glass swan and drank a fair amount. I passed the bird to Steph as if we were sharing a glass of milk, and she drank the liquid also. Once again, I had succeeded in making yet another friend my accomplice in mischief. Steph should have refused my invitation, but she didn't. With my crazy ideas, anyone was better off not listening to me.

The weather bird was no more.

Steph and I made our way back downstairs, and Steph decided to tell our parents what we had done. She didn't have to say a word; our blue tongues betrayed us. Panic seized my mom and the rest of the family. It was time for another call to the poison control center. My mom was gaining knowledge of poison control, so she knew she had to call because different poisons require different antidotes. It was too bad we didn't have speed dial in the 1980s because my mom really could have used it.

I guess I should have known what was coming, but I didn't really think ahead much, if you hadn't noticed. Not only had I endangered my own life once again, I had also endangered someone else's.

After Mom's conversation with the poison control center, she mixed up the life-saving concoction of milk and ipecac. Steph and I cringed at the thought of drinking the nasty liquid, but our parents gave us no choice. I knew from past experience that it wasn't pleasant. We drank it down, vomiting commenced, and play ceased. We both felt terribly sick. Having our own weatherman was not as fun as I thought it would be.

Surely now I had learned my lesson. Yeah right! A few years later at the white house, I chugged a bottle of Avon Bird of Paradise perfume. Maybe I just had an obsession with birds. I don't know. At least this time I only took myself down. I had mercy upon all my friends and family.

I can still taste that perfume to this day if I think about it. Words cannot describe the terrible flavor. It was a taste I thought would never leave my mouth.

My mom was ready though. By then she had the poison control center's number memorized. For safety's sake she called, but she already knew what to do. Consequently, she was calmer as she headed for the kitchen to mix my favorite drink. I was filled with dread when I considered what the drink would do to me. It was a terrible thought that I did not want to become a reality. Mom handed me the drink and I tried not to gag as I sent it down my throat. I would again endure the sickness that followed. Fortunately, this would be the last time I consumed something poisonous. Finally, I had learned from my mistakes and my sickness.

Chapter 11

A New Day

Dr. Wood arrived the morning of my fourth day in the hospital.

"Your ultrasound came back good," he said. "There doesn't seem to be any problem in your legs, and the X-ray looked good. I think the pain in your legs will gradually get better, but I'm not sure what is causing it."

"That sounds good," I said.

"You should be able to go home tomorrow," he added.

"Great," I replied.

I was excited about going home. Four days in a hospital does little for one's self-image. I had not bathed, brushed my teeth, or combed my hair. There was a suspicious odor in my room, and I was coming to accept that it was me.

Hygiene becomes less a priority when you have forty staples, numerous patches of sticky tape, and a tube running out your back.

"We're going to take your tube out today," Dr. Wood said.

I nodded okay. Dr. Wood and Justin made small talk for a moment, and then Dr. Wood left the room.

"How is that tube staying in place in my back?" I asked Justin.

He looked at me nervously and said, "They sewed it to your skin."

Ignorance is bliss. I should have learned that by now.

"Yuck," I replied, making a face.

The thought of that tube being sewn into my skin sent a wave of nausea to my stomach.

Fortunately, I was able to rest the remainder of the morning. Around lunchtime, the physical therapist came, and I was ready for my workout. The expectation of going home, coupled with a restful morning, had energized me. I felt that God was truly renewing my strength, and I knew He would continue to strengthen me and give me peace. "The Lord gives strength to his people; The Lord blesses his people with peace" (Psalm 29:11 NIV). I slowly made my way out of the bed with help and placed my hands on the walker. We strolled out the door and down the hall.

"I want to see how you do on the steps," the PT said.

"Okay," I said.

We made our way to the stairwell at the end of the hall. As I looked out the glass windows I once again felt hope surge within me. Tomorrow I would breathe the fresh air and feel a breeze on my face. I didn't care if it *was* February and the breeze might be below freezing; I just wanted to feel the outdoors again. Oh, how I cherished the view from those windows and the hope it provided!

We entered the stairwell, and my PT held my right arm as I grasped the rail to my left. Justin was very close to me in case I needed help. I went up the steps at a tortoise-like pace—slow but sure.

"You're doing well," said my PT. "Let's see if you can go down the steps now."

"Okay," I said as I turned and headed back down the steps.

"Good job," she said. "I think you'll be fine when you get home."

The physical therapist had taken me to their office and workout room the day before, and I had made it up a couple of steps, but now I was able to do even more. We have four steps in our home; she wanted me to be able to climb at least four so I would have confidence in getting around at our house. I still needed help, but I was getting better each day. I found this progress encouraging. It gave me hope for the days ahead.

"Let's head back to your room," she said.

As we made our way back I asked to walk a little more, so we circled the nurses' station before returning to my room.

"I hear you're going home soon," my PT said.

"Yes!" I said joyfully.

"I'm sure you can't wait," she said.

I nodded. I couldn't wait, and I wanted to express it, but the exertion had sapped my energy. To converse would require more energy than I had left. She helped me back into bed and walked out the door. My nurse entered shortly after.

"You need to push your morphine pump a couple of times," she said. "We're going to remove the tube from your back."

Too exhausted to argue, I followed her instructions and tried to rest.

"Is that going to hurt?" I asked.

She looked at me a little funny, as if to say "of course it hurts." Instead, she said, "You need to push your morphine button as much as it will let you until I get back."

I lay there trying to regain my strength. My mind started tossing around the thought of getting that tube pulled out of my back. This sounded intense, but I figured it was something I had to do to get out of the hospital. Dread filled me, but there was nothing I could do but take it. Asking for anesthesia would be a lost cause.

After about fifteen minutes my nurse came back to remove the drain tube. As she flipped on her latex gloves, queasiness filled my stomach; I knew this was going to be bad.

"Roll over on your side," she said.

Justin came over to give me a hand to squeeze. I could feel my nurse clipping the stitches that ran through my skin.

"You need to take a deep breath," she said.

I inhaled deeply, and as I did she quickly pulled the tube from my back. Justin could see the whole process, but I was relieved that my view was blocked. Yes, it was painful, but it was over quickly. I must say my nurse did an excellent job. I didn't even know she was going to pull the tube when I took the deep breath. Because of that, I didn't have the opportunity to get even more nervous. I now had another obstacle behind me.

Television, rest, and visitors consumed the rest of my day. Belle and her husband Mike came by as well as some of my former WKU coaches and their families. The support was uplifting and the visits comforting.

The next morning I awoke to my favorite person. I was on the verge of asking her not to draw my blood, but instead I chanted in my mind "this is the last time, this is the last time," over and over until she was done. I'm not sure why I just didn't refuse them drawing my blood, but I never did.

Dr. Wood came in early that morning.

"You ready to go home?" he said.

I nodded and gave a wide smile.

"We'll get your IV out and get you on your way," he said. "The nurse will give you some instructions on what you can and can't do. Your pain should get better all the time. You're doing great."

"Thank you," I said as he exited.

My nurse came in and told me I could change into my own clothes. I was elated to hear this—finally some clothes that did not expose my whole backside. I felt a twinge of concern over the actual process of changing clothes. I knew it would be exhausting and challenging, but Justin was able to help me, and I was ready to move forward. After getting dressed, it was time for my last physical therapy session, at least in the hospital. Once again we walked down the hall toward the big windows. As I looked out through the glass, I knew I would soon be out there with the air and the trees. That was exciting.

We walked down other halls of the hospital. I walked more that day than I had before. It felt good, but my therapist and I decided I should save some energy for the trip home. As I rounded the nurses' station and returned to my room, my anticipation grew. I was getting closer to home with every minute. The tube was gone, I was wearing my own clothes, and I had completed my last physical therapy session in the hospital. Now I needed the IV removed and I was on my way.

Soon my nurse arrived to take out the IV. I was glad to get that thing out. After five days, it was really starting to burn whenever they gave me meds through it. I had asked each nurse to go slowly when they put medication in it because the burning sensation was very painful. They all complied with my requests. I was starting to think I needed a morphine pump just to get my IV meds.

Belle had arrived to help us pack and get home. She would pick up my prescriptions so that Justin could take me directly home. She truly was a blessing during my hospital stay. Belle and Justin scurried around gathering my things and making sure nothing was left behind. I lay still watching the entire action take place, waiting for my cue to exit.

Finally my driver arrived with my wheelchair, and it was time for me to say goodbye. He wheeled me down to the nurses' station. I thanked them for caring for me. Each nurse had provided for my needs exceptionally. We then went down the elevator and reached the front door. Justin ran ahead to get our vehicle. As we exited the hospital I inhaled deeply and breathed in the fresh air. I had dreamed of this moment every time I looked out those glass windows during therapy. Now it was here. I had been through so much, but now I had made it out.

Justin and my wheelchair driver helped me into the car, and we were on our way. Every bump and turn hurt. I can't say I enjoyed the ride. I was dizzy and nauseated, and I had to strain to keep my body still during the turns. After the long drive, we finally arrived home. Belle, who had gone ahead of us, was waiting. Justin helped me out of the car, and with

Belle on one arm and a cane in the other hand, I made baby steps to the back door.

Here I was, all 185 pounds of me, putting my entire weight in the hands of 5-foot-nothing Belle and a sturdy stick. If I fell, Belle was supposed to catch me. What were we thinking? I inched forward, holding onto Belle for dear life. Justin unlocked the door and made a place for me to lie down. I inched along, but finally, with Belle still by my side, I reached the couch. Our couch is low, so it would take both Justin and Belle to get me down to it. As I let go of my weight on the pillows I felt a rush of exhaustion overwhelm me.

I rested a bit as Justin and Belle made ready everything I might need. I then managed to get in the shower. We have a shower with a seat in it that is somewhat handicap accessible. With some help, I was able to get rid of most of the stench. Justin washed my hair and Belle dried it. Every move I made sent pain into my back, so I had to be careful. With their assistance, I made my way back to the couch and didn't move anymore unless I needed to go to the bathroom. Words cannot express how exhausted I was.

A lot of things changed during my five days in the hospital. I went into the hospital able to walk on my own and left needing both a cane and another person to support me. I went in the hospital with a little pride, and I left every bit of it inside those doors. I went in smelling clean, and when I left a stench followed behind me like Pigpen in the Charlie Brown comic strip. I experienced both utter humility and great joy, not to mention an abundance of emotions in between. I had finally made my way out of the hospital and through my back door. God had protected me, held me, comforted me, and brought me this far. "Fear not, for I have redeemed you; I have called you by your name; You are mine. When you pass through the waters, I will be with you; and through the rivers, they shall not overflow you. When you walk through the fire, you shall not be burned, nor shall the flame scorch you" (Isaiah 43:1-2 NKJV).

Chapter 12

Trampoline

I always had an obsession for jumping. When I was younger, I regularly jumped my bike off our porch at the white house. I would build ramps with cement blocks and wood to jump off of. The higher the ramps, the better. I was always looking for a new way to fly, if only for a moment. Jumping tempted me the way most kids are tempted by candy; I could not resist. As a result, I probably have more jumping stories than anyone would care to hear.

As I reached my teenage years, not a whole lot had changed. I was the same energetic thrill-seeker, except now I could drive. It goes without saying that I often caused my parents to worry. They started a prayer chain every time I left the house.

In high school, I had a group of friends I was very close to, and we all hung out together; other times we ran in smaller groups. On this particular sunny day, Christi and I were spending time together at her house, a one-story ranch house with a big yard and a sidewalk leading up to the front door.

Christi's brother owned a trampoline. My parents never would have bought me a trampoline—a wise decision on their part. I remember the trampoline catching my attention as we walked up the sidewalk. As I eyed it thoughts rolled through my mind. I was thinking of how much fun it would be to give it a try. Christi and I went inside, and I successfully put all thoughts about the trampoline aside for a while.

As time passed, Christi and I returned outside, and my preoccupation with the trampoline resumed. Gazing at it, I got a brilliant idea. I thought it would be fun to really test the trampoline. I decided to climb onto the roof of Christi's house and take a leap onto the trampoline. This would achieve a much longer time of flight than just jumping on it normally. I shared my thoughts with Christi.

"You're crazy," she said.

She was probably correct, but I didn't care. Christi's brother, Blake, was at home and he thought I had a good idea, so he decided to join me. We started our climb to the rooftop by way of a four-wheeler and a windowsill. In a matter of seconds we reached our destination. My adrenaline was pumping and I was ready to take the leap. My stomach had moved into my throat. I loved that feeling of excitement and uncertainty.

I didn't calculate how far I needed to jump. I didn't think about how high I might rebound after I made contact with the trampoline. I didn't think about anything. I just leapt off the roof onto the trampoline. In that brief moment, I felt the exhilaration of air whizzing by my body; it was a wonderful feeling. I was flying, even if only for a second. But then SMACK! I hit the trampoline. I felt the air flowing past me and the flying sensation again. I did it! I had managed to jump off the roof, hit the trampoline, and survive without injury. Blake had also done the same. We had pushed the limits of the trampoline and lived.

This was fun to me. I liked the rush that came with it, looking fear in the face. I liked pushing the limits. Sometimes, I admit, I pushed *past* the limits, but I was glad I didn't let fear stop me from doing things. I'm sure my parents weren't happy with all my decisions, but it was who I was. I enjoyed smiling at the fear and moving forward as if it didn't exist.

The jump from the roof to the trampoline was so exciting I climbed back up and made my way off the roof again. There we were defying gravity, if only for a brief moment. Christi stood aside and watched, choosing not to put her body in harm's way, shaking her head with every jump. It was a good thing my friends made wiser choices than I did. I could have been persuaded to do about anything. Luckily, I had calm friends who didn't really want to push the limits. If I had been friends with other daredevils like myself, it would have undoubtedly meant more trouble and probably severe injuries to one or all of us.

Chapter 13

Home

As I began my recovery at home, I was completely dependent on others. I needed care from sunup to sundown. I could do very little by myself. I needed someone to get me out of bed and someone to put me into bed. I needed someone to give me a shower and fix my meals. I was a full-time job for Justin.

Upon my departure from the hospital, I received some literature regarding my recovery. It included a list of do's and don'ts, as well as what to do if a fever developed or a rash appeared. As I looked over the list I began to wonder what I could do. The list included rules such as: don't sit for over ten minutes, don't bend at the waist, don't drive, and so on. I had to accept that most of my time would be spent on the couch or in the bed, at least for a few weeks.

For the first few days, I was so fatigued I just wanted to lie there. I would stare at the ceiling or the wall, unable even to focus on a TV show. After the first few days, I started to feel like I could watch TV or read, which was nice. My days were all the same; it felt as if I were in the movie *Groundhog Day*. I would wake up and call Justin to come get me out of bed. I moaned with each movement of my back, which at this point was any movement at all. Justin would pull me out of bed and help me to the bathroom to get ready for the day. I would then drag my feet to the living room and hit the couch for the day. After my breakfast I would watch ESPN's *Sportscenter* to catch up on all the sporting news. Just the morning ritual and the trip to the couch were enough to exhaust me. I was amazed that so little exertion required all my energy.

There's not a whole lot you can do on the couch. I learned that quickly. I read five books during my recovery time and watched more movies than I care to admit. I wrote some, I cried some, and I went stir-crazy some. Even though I didn't feel well enough to go outside yet, nonetheless I experienced "cabin fever" on a regular basis. Visitors came occasionally, and that helped to pass the time and break up the monotony of repetitive days. Otherwise, I did what I could to pass the time.

Walking was on the doctor's "do" list, so I walked as much as I could. With Justin on one arm and my cane in the other hand, I made circles in our living room and walked until I was too tired to keep going. After about four days at home, I decided to venture outside. Every other day I went out to walk. When I first got home I had set a goal to walk down our driveway, which is about a quarter-mile long. I believed this to be a lofty but attainable goal.

The dogs were always happy to see me come outside. On one particular day they got a little too excited and bumped into me. Fortunately, I braced myself and no harm was done. Still, it's scary having two big dogs coming at you when you have the speed, agility, and balance of a baby.

I most looked forward to the walks outside. Unfortunately, if I were walking, someone had to be with me. I didn't make it very far at first, but each time I walked a few steps farther. After my walk my energy was so diminished I could barely get through a shower and back on the couch. When the fatigue overwhelmed me, I questioned how I ever got to that point. To make things worse, I was still fighting the pain in my legs. This just discouraged me further. What kind of weakling had I become? I pondered this often.

After my surgery, my life changed a lot. I was trying to get off the pain medications and back to a somewhat normal life. I was trying to learn how to live again. I was trying to learn to walk on my own again. I was trying to do a lot, but most importantly I was trying to learn who I was. I had always considered myself a strong, active person, someone who helped others, not someone who needed others for help. I was learning to be humble. I was learning to let others do almost everything for me.

I didn't want to be dependent on others, but now that was my situation. Everything had changed in my life, and I had to adjust to that. Even though I didn't want to be dependent on others, I could feel God's presence so strongly in my life because of my brokenness. "So we fix our eyes not on what is seen, but on what is unseen. For what is seen is temporary, but what is unseen is eternal" (2 Corinthians 4:18 NIV). Although I could not see God right there with me, I knew He was there and that I needed to focus on Him and not my situation. I felt Him around me now as I never had before.

It was discouraging to be unable to do the things I could before, but I had to believe that God still had a great purpose for me. I had been an athlete. I had been strong. I had been self-sufficient. All those things were no more. I took pride in my accomplishments, but now those accomplishments seemed so far away. I left my pride at the hospital, and humility was becoming a daily lesson—one I would not have chosen, but God was speaking to me through it and because of it. I was so grateful now for each chore done for me. I was more thankful in my heart than I had ever been. Each display of love touched my life in such a special way. These displays of love would not have occurred had I not been so broken.

Also, as I became incapable I realized how capable God was. Although I could do nothing, He could do all things. He was my protector, my hope, and my guide. "The Lord is my rock and my fortress and my deliverer. The God of my strength, in whom I will trust" (2 Samuel 22:2 NKJV). I am so thankful for God's tangible presence during those difficult days. I had to believe my worth hadn't left me when my skills and agility did. I had to keep hope that I would heal and be able to do something in this life that I would want to do and that would matter.

I combated discouragement and boredom by walking. My few steps had turned into a few more steps, and I was getting closer to the end of the driveway, little by little. Six days after coming home, I made it a third of the way down our driveway. We have a pond about that far from our house, and I enjoyed seeing the water. I was so elated to make it to the pond. It was amazing how once-trivial accomplishments had become such major milestones. When I first got home, I could only walk about twenty yards at a time. I tried to go a little farther each day, whether inside or out. As I walked outside, I took deep breaths to soak up the fresh air. I listened to the birds singing their sweet melodies, reminding me of the renewal of the coming spring. On a really good day, my horses would come near so I could pet them. Seeing the horses always brightened my day, and I think it brightened theirs too.

Whenever I walked, I had to wear my brace. Oh, what a brace it was! It was molded specifically to fit my body. The hard plastic brace could be compared to a 17th-century corset. It wrapped around my upper body from my hipbones to under my arms. To say that it was uncomfortable would be an understatement. If it was fastened too tight, I could hardly breathe. Justin, in his diligence and wanting me to heal properly, sometimes cut my air a little short as he squeezed the brace to get it very snug. I managed, but I hated the brace.

No Fear

The longer I wore it, the more I hated it. Hate is a harsh word, but here it is absolutely appropriate.

Each day I felt stronger. My body was slowly healing. I was learning to get up more on my own, but not totally by myself yet. I could walk a bit faster. I did a little more each day, but it was slow going. When Dr. Wood first told me I would have to take off work for two or three months, I thought he was crazy. Now I knew, as I faced each new day, that it would take at least that long and maybe even longer for me to feel normal again.

Chapter 14

Trouble

I didn't really like school as a kid. I didn't really like school *anytime*. It just wasn't my thing. I did okay in school, but I didn't enjoy it. There's something about having to sit still for hours at a time that just doesn't mesh with my personality. I wanted to be moving and doing something adventurous all the time. I did love playing basketball though. Basketball is what kept me focused enough to pass in school. In fact, I owned a T-shirt in high school that clearly illustrated my attitude. It read, "If it wasn't for basketball, I'd quit school." Indeed, I might have quit school anyway if I didn't have such caring parents.

In elementary school, I found my niche on the McKee Bulldogs girls' basketball team. I began playing on the fifth and sixth grade team with my friend Misti when we were in second grade. We held down the bench, but we enjoyed watching the games and got to play in practice. In short, we had fun.

We continued to play on the team as we grew older, and we both enjoyed every moment of it. Misti was multitalented: she would play in the games, do a quick Superman-like change of uniform, and run out at halftime with the dance team. When the horn announced the end of halftime, she would be right back in her basketball uniform and ready to resume play.

Our basketball coach was also my English teacher. As class was ending one day, he asked me to go and retrieve our uniforms from his truck. He had taken them home to wash them, and they needed to be brought in for our next game. I happily obliged. Any excuse to go outside was a good one. I headed out the classroom door and straight to the parking lot. He didn't give me his keys because no one locked their doors in McKee, Kentucky, in those days. Things were good and locks usually weren't needed.

I opened the door to the Dodge Ram and peered inside. What I found there surprised me. In the truck I found a loaded pistol! Normally I would have had no interest in the gun, but the Sunday before, Dad had taken his pistol to my grandparents' farm to do some shooting. Since I wanted to be involved in everything, I tagged along. He explained to me how the gun worked and talked about gun safety. He even allowed me to shoot his gun a couple of times. I had a good time that Sunday with my dad. As a result, I was intrigued.

So there I was with a pistol before me. I guess it's evident by now that I didn't always make the best decisions. A "good kid" would have bypassed the gun and done her job, but Coach didn't send the "good kid." He sent me. I picked up the gun and looked through the sights. I put my finger on the trigger, imagining the cowboys in the movies. Before I knew it, there was an ear-popping BOOM! I had applied enough pressure to move the trigger, and BANG! the gun went off. I was scared to death. My mind ran wild as to what I should do. The gun had blown a hole in the passenger-side door of the truck. Terrified of getting in trouble, I grabbed the uniforms and quietly made my way back into the school.

I dropped the uniforms off in the gym and immediately went to get Misti out of class. I needed someone to talk to and get advice from. I told Misti what had just happened.

"What am I supposed to do?" I asked her frantically.

You can imagine the look on her face. I had just told her I shot a hole in our coach's truck! She didn't know what to tell me. At this point we were confused, scared, and overwhelmed. I hastily devised a plan. It was ludicrous, but I was desperate. I would lie.

I went back to my English class to talk with my coach.

"I heard a noise like a gunshot coming from the apartments," I said.

There were some apartment buildings very near to the school, and I decided that would be my best choice for placing the blame. I did not consider the important fact that if a gun were shot from the apartments it would have hit the tailgate or the back window of the truck, not the passenger door. It was also obvious that the shot came from inside the truck rather than outside it. Though this happened years before *CSI* premiered, it did not require a genius to figure out the details. I acted out of panic.

"I'm not sure what happened," I said. "It sounded like somebody from the apartments shot a gun."

He looked at me surprised and confused. I continued with my fabricated story, but it in no way helped the situation. After I spoke with him, my coach went outside to his truck to investigate. It was now obvious I was lying. I was in big trouble.

He called my parents, and the gig was up for me. I finally admitted what I had done. To say it was embarrassing would be putting it lightly. I knew what I did was wrong, and I knew this would be the talk of our small town for awhile. Not only had I shot the truck, but I had also tried to cover everything up with ridiculous lies. This was different from my other antics because I had done something I knew was morally unacceptable. I had managed to get myself into a terrible ordeal. I was very fortunate not to have hurt myself or someone else.

I had been saving my extra money for a few years to buy a four-wheeler. I wanted one so badly. Because of my actions, my four-wheeler savings went toward fixing a gunshot hole in a red Dodge Ram. I also paid in other ways. There was punishment from my parents and criticism from others. A few days later, a woman I'd known for most of my life came up to me with her arms in the air and said, "You're not going to shoot me, are you?"

I will never forget that. Her words flooded me with feelings of hurt and embarrassment. The situation was already difficult for me, and her insensitive joke simply intensified my shame and added insult to injury. Even now I can close my eyes and relive the incident, feeling humiliation wash over me.

Chapter 15

Checkup

As previously mentioned, anytime I left the house Mr. Brace was right by my side, literally. This was one of the "do's" on Dr. Wood's list that I could "do" without. It was time for my first checkup since leaving the hospital, and I knew it would be an adventure. Mr. Brace and I boarded the vehicle with Justin's help. Once the car was moving, I had to hold on with both my hands and feet, as any bump would send pain through my back. Down the road we went back to the place that got me into this mess. We arrived on time, and I was ready to get checked out and go back home. Justin and I sat patiently in the waiting room.

"Shea," the nurse called. It was my turn.

No Fear

Yes, the brace was very uncomfortable, but have I mentioned how hot it was? I could break a sweat in ten seconds flat after putting it on. As we sat in the doctor's office, I could feel beads of sweat sliding down my back and stomach. Though it felt disgusting, I couldn't take the brace off. Can you imagine?

I considered the alternative. "Hey, Dr. Wood, here I am not wearing my brace after only two weeks. Just thought I would carry it with me instead. You don't mind, right?"

Sweaty or not, I didn't think taking the brace off would sit well with my doctor, so I sucked it up and sweated off a few pounds. On the bright side, sweating was a good start at shedding the twenty or so pounds I had packed on while becoming close companions with our couch.

After about twenty minutes, Dr. Wood came into the room.

"How are you?" he asked.

"I'm doing good," I said. "A bit hot."

"Yes, those braces can be pretty warm," he said nonchalantly.

You're telling me, I thought. He asked me to remove the brace, and I was elated. He wanted to examine my back to see how it was healing.

"Everything looks good," he said. "I'm going to take out half of your staples today."

I had often worried about the staple removal. Lying on my couch, I contemplated the pain I might feel as the staples pulled out. I had heard from others that it was bad, so I was prepared for the worst.

I leaned over the table, my body tensing in apprehension. The doctor started working his way down my back pulling out every other staple. It hurt, of course, but the pain was tolerable. With the removal of each staple, I felt a burning sensation. Fortunately, Dr. Wood's skillful hands worked quickly, and he adeptly dislodged half the staples in a matter of seconds. By this time I had nearly weaned myself from the pain medicine, so I could feel the stinging acutely, but it could have been worse.

Afterwards, Justin helped me get my brace back on, and I sat down. Dr. Wood asked me if I had any more questions.

"Can I stay at home by myself?" I asked.

"Yes, that will be fine," he said.

I shot Justin a glance because I knew he didn't want to leave me alone. I could tell by the surprised look on his face that he didn't expect Dr. Wood to say yes. He was afraid I would fall or not be able to get things I needed. I was excited about this news, but I wasn't sure I could convince Justin to leave me even with Dr. Wood's approval. Justin had become more protective of me after seeing me so broken and dependent on others.

At this point I was just ready to get out of that office. I was feeling more and more tired and in need of a place to rest a little. I had my first checkup behind me, short and sweaty.

Justin and I headed out the door on our way home, or so *he* thought. In my "infinite wisdom" I decided that I should visit Mike and Belle. I wanted to show them how far I had come. I particularly wanted Belle to see how much better I could walk and how much more I could do for myself.

"Are you sure that's a good idea?" Justin said. "I don't think you're ready for that much."

"Yeah, I'll be okay," I said.

"That's a lot for your first time away from the house since being released from the hospital."

"I think I'll be fine," I insisted, and on we went.

We arrived at Mike and Belle's house to their surprise. I wasn't ready for all this action, but I thought I could do it. Justin and I visited with them for about twenty minutes and told them all about my appointment. I had my brace on, so I couldn't lie down or sit comfortably. As a result, I got more and more fatigued. The brace made my spine completely straight. With it on, I had perfect posture, but it was tiring and uncomfortable to sit perched like a bird. I knew I needed to go home.

"We need to be going," I said. "I'm going to have to lie down."

"Let's go then," Justin said.

He helped me up, and we slowly made our way to the door with the help of my cane. He lowered me into our vehicle and went to the other side to get in. I braced myself by holding onto the door with one hand and the console with the other. I also put both feet all the way forward and pushed them against the floorboard. I was now ready for the drive. I desperately needed to lie down and rest.

Back at home, the rest of the day was typical. I rested, ate, and took a shower. I was exhausted from the day's events. That night I started feeling very ill and asked Justin to help me to bed early. As I lay in bed, my body started shaking, and I was overcome with cold sweats. I became nauseated. Vomiting would be very painful, so I wanted to avoid that. I lay there for about an hour shaking and sweating with the trashcan beside the bed. Had I caught something at the doctor's office? I lay there praying for relief. After about an hour I decided to try to sleep, hoping that morning would bring a better day. I fell asleep and awoke the next morning feeling better. When I told family members what had happened the night before, the consensus was that I had overdone things and made myself sick. I knew I was tired, but I didn't think I was *that* tired. That is what I reaped for relying on my own wisdom instead of listening to the godly wisdom of my husband.

In the meantime, I was getting around better each day. I had become strong enough to get myself up off the couch. I could use my arms to raise my upper body to a sitting position. As my upper body rose up, my legs were supposed to lower at the same time so that I stayed straight. After making it to the sitting position, I could use the armrest and my cane to push off the floor and reach a standing position.

The cane also enabled me to use the bathroom on my own. Days before, Justin had to help me sit down and get up from the toilet as well as wash my hands since I couldn't lean over the sink. Now I could use my cane to lower myself and to get up. Justin filled a cup with water and left it sitting by the sink so I could use that water to rinse my hands. It was a big cup, so it would last me most of the day. This arrangement allowed me to use the bathroom alone again.

It only got ugly when I dropped my cane. Since I could not bend, it was a challenge to get the cane back in my hands. I had received a grabber in the hospital so I wouldn't have to bend to reach things. At first I was not proficient in using the grabber, so picking up the cane could be a challenge. Also, if the grabber was in another room, I tried to scoot the cane up a wall with my feet. It took me a few minutes sometimes, but I would eventually recover the cane. The cane and grabber had restored some of my independence since they allowed me to reach places and do things I previously relied on others to do.

I was inching down the long road of recovery. I had learned to do more on my own, including activities that just a few days earlier were impossible. I could feel myself getting stronger and knew I was slowly healing. As days passed, I began to see more clearly a vision for a "normal" future. I often thought of playing basketball and doing other activities I had enjoyed so much before. I was fairly certain my life would not be the same, but as I recovered I had hope for my future. "Praise be to the Lord, for he has heard my cry for mercy. The Lord is my strength and my shield; my heart trusts in him and I am helped. My heart leaps for joy and I will give thanks to him in song" (Psalm 28:6-7 NIV).

Chapter 16

Learning to Drive

The Cole Oil Company bulk plant was a place of excitement and adventure when I was growing up. Everyone had to stay alert, as accidents were known to occur from time to time. I had run through a glass door at the plant, and my cousin Stephanie had fallen off a stack of boxes of oil when we were playing on them. She had to be rushed to the local doctor because she was bleeding so much. They stitched her up, but she still has the scar from that accident. There was always something going on. Looking back, I can't help wondering how any work ever got accomplished.

I was at the plant almost on a daily basis. On occasion my cousins from Waco would come and visit us. These cousins were my mom's sister, Trish's, kids: Andrew, Hannah, and

Matthew. I looked forward to their visits. I was older than all of them, so I introduced them to all the fun things they didn't have in Waco and showed them the ropes. Andrew was the oldest. One summer he came to Jackson County to spend some quality time with his Aunt Betty Lou, his Uncle Larry, and his elder cousin Shea. Trish was entrusting the care of her firstborn to the Lunsfords.

I had "learned"—and I use the word lightly—to drive at a young age. My dad owned a little Ford Courier truck, and I could drive around the fields by our house. Sometimes I was allowed to drive at the plant. The truck was a stick shift, so I had my fair share of hopping and jumping whenever I started and stopped. I've definitely ground out a few gears in my time. I had trails beaten down in the fields by our house and a path I always followed that was in the gate, down and up the hill, around the pond, and so on. I loved driving in our fields. I felt so grown up. I would wave at the passersby with my chin up.

It was a weekday, so my mom had to work. This meant that Andrew and I would be spending some time at the bulk plant. There were so many things for us to do! I did not even know where to begin. We could climb on some cases of oil, go play in the creek, or figure out some practical joke to play on Cleva or one of the other unsuspecting employees. So much to do, and so little time.

In an effort to show Andrew just how big I was and what I was capable of doing, I chose for us to take a ride in my dad's truck. By now I considered myself an expert, and I was ready to showcase my skills to my younger cousin.

I can't remember whether I asked permission to take the truck. Perhaps I assumed it was all right. In Jackson County people left their vehicles unlocked, and they sometimes even left the keys in the ignition. That's how things worked; I figured if the door was unlocked and the keys were inside it was an invitation to drive the Courier.

"You want to go for a ride?" I asked, a mischievous sparkle in my eyes.

"Yeah, let's go," Andrew said.

He's ready to watch his big cousin in action, I thought. *He's ready to learn the ropes of driving, and who better to teach him than me?*

We started toward the truck, and both of us jumped in. I could see the excitement in his face, and I was excited to show him how much I could do. I started up the truck and backed away from the small loading dock. There were two loading docks at the plant, one to load boxes, drums of oil, and other such products. The second, larger dock was used for loading our gas trucks for their deliveries. If you walked out the plant office, you would be on the small loading dock, and most people parked near the edge of the smaller dock when they were going inside the office. There was also a stockroom up on the small dock. The larger dock for the trucks was a little farther away, but you could walk to it. Between the two docks was gravel where I could drive back and forth when we didn't have customers. There was also a small field behind the plant and a large creek behind the field. I had plenty of space to drive my dad's truck.

Andrew and I had begun our journey, and we were having a blast. The radio roared, and we felt as free as the wind and bigger than ever. We must have been the envy of every child around. We made our way up and down the drive around the plant, the breeze blowing our hair. After a few trips up and down the drive, I decided to park the truck and go in the office to see if anything new and exciting was going on.

I started to ease down to the loading dock to put my dad's truck back where it was before. We got closer, and it was time for me to hit the brakes and start slowing us to a stop. As I reached for the brake my foot ended up on the gas instead. We smashed straight into the loading dock. I knew immediately that I was in serious trouble again. I wondered if Andrew was okay. I looked over and he was in tears. He fumbled for the door handle, trying to get out of the truck. I think he just wanted to get as far away from me and the truck as possible. Instead of showing him a good time, I had traumatized him. As he ran for the office door, I wondered if he would ever be the same.

My thoughts raced. What should I do? I matched Andrew's sprint with slow steps. With each step, my apprehension gained momentum. I examined the front of the truck and my stomach leaped into my throat. Sure enough, the impact had damaged the front of the truck. Surely swift punishment awaited me. This was my dad's truck, the parent I did not dare cross. I made sure he was not around when plotting such adventures as jumping off the church balcony. He was a wonderful father who certainly believed in discipline. He also had a bit of a temper. I knew I would incur his wrath when he saw the damage to his truck.

I could no longer avoid the inevitable; I had to go inside. By now everyone must know. When Andrew ran into the office in tears, everyone would have asked him why he was crying. I started inside with my head lowered. My dad was

No Fear

not there at the moment, but I knew he would find out. There was no way of hiding the busted front end of his truck.

As I entered, I saw my mom consoling Andrew. I sat down on the couch and waited my turn. Mom had already phoned my dad. She said he would be there soon after he got off work. I was in hot water. I didn't move from the couch. Likewise, a still shaken Andrew didn't leave my mom's side.

Time slowly passed as I anticipated my dad's entrance. Suddenly, the door opened and he appeared. I knew a severe spanking was in my future. I knew some of my privileges would be revoked. I dreaded what awaited me. But what I thought was coming did not actually occur. My dad, after seeing that Andrew and I were so shaken up, chose to let this be a lesson learned. He knew I was scared by the situation, and because of this I avoided punishment. I did learn a valuable lesson though from the forgiving, loving spirit of my father.

Andrew also learned a lesson: don't ride in any vehicles with Shea! It would be years before he got in a vehicle with me behind the wheel. I thought of these lessons each time I passed by the front end of the Ford Courier.

Chapter 17

Healing

Three weeks after my surgery, I was able to stay at home alone. All the more reason for fear to try to creep into my mind. Fear is everywhere. We pretend it's not, but it is. Almost everyone is afraid of something, yet we praise and glorify the man who says he fears nothing. We put him on TV and make an idol out of him. We exalt the one who is not afraid to drive a bike off a cliff or who plays "chicken" with the oncoming driver. We idolize people who say they live without fear. A company has even branded the term "No Fear." But fear lives on, whether we admit it or not. We don't really want to talk about it, but it is there, like a predator hiding in the darkness, waiting to overwhelm its next victim.

As I lay at home alone, I prayed I would not become fear's next victim.

What did I fear? I feared not being able to do things I once did. I feared a life of pain. I feared not functioning normally again. Knowing that fear is not in God's plan, I reigned over it by recalling the words of Isaiah 41:10, "Fear not, for I am with you" (NKJV). I realized that I was not alone. In the presence of God, fear flees. In three weeks He had brought me so far, and I knew He had more great things in store for me. I clung to that hope and to the wonderful things God had done for me. "But those who hope in the Lord will renew their strength. They will soar on wings like eagles; they will run and not grow weary, they will walk and not be faint" (Isaiah 40:31 NIV).

I am comforted by such verses and gain strength from them. They are wonderful words of hope for God's people to cling to.

It was time for lunch, my first lunch alone. Justin had my food prepared; all I had to do was put it on a plate and heat it in the microwave. In all my life, I never thought heating up lunch would be a challenge, especially at the age of thirty-one.

I was able to get my first serving heated without any problems. I sat down to eat, and thanksgiving flowed from my heart. I ate my leftovers and decided I would like something else. I reassured myself that a healing body must need seconds. The food I wanted was in the bottom drawer of our refrigerator. Keep in mind, I still could not bend at the waist. After movements that would win a championship game of Twister, I achieved success; finally I had reached the tomatoes and fresh mozzarella.

As I began to dice the tomatoes, I started shaking. At the same time my coordination left me, and it was all I could do to get the tomatoes cut. I was shaking from the fatigue of getting out of the chair, retrieving a tomato and some cheese, and cutting it up. Could this be real? It seemed only a short time since I could play an entire game of basketball without any shaking. And now I was cutting a tomato and about to pass out. *This can't be real!* I thought.

"Will this ever get better?" I said aloud.

There it was again—fear. I believe the devil seizes any opportunity to creep into our thoughts. He waits for his chance, and my shaking and childlike coordination gave it to him. When someone's health deteriorates, as mine had, our vulnerability increases, affording Satan optimal opportunities to shoot his arrows of fear. What was my defense? I tried to keep centered on God and His Word, but it was hard. I remembered that "perfect love casts out fear" and that God is perfect love. I stopped and asked for God's help through a silent prayer.

Finally, through answered prayers, the tremors subsided and I was able to finish chopping the tomatoes. I tossed them into a bowl with the mozzarella and headed down the stairs to finish my meal. As I watched the last few bites disappear, I silently retorted that maybe a healing body does not need seconds, but rather to hit the couch after the first serving. I would keep that in mind for the future.

After lunch, it was time to lie down again. Fatigue drew me to the couch. As I walked down the four steps to the living room, I bypassed the couch and walked over to our double patio doors. The sun was beaming in and felt warm to my face. I closed my eyes, and in that moment I felt a gentle touch run across my face. I imagined it was God's touch, and I remembered that He never leaves us. I felt very alone that day, but I was not alone. God had carried me through. He had calmed me, reassured me, and never left me.

"Thank You, Lord, for the warmth of the sunshine and the warmth of Your love that casts out my fears," I said.

Chapter 18

Four-Wheelin'

Charles was my first boyfriend, if you can call someone you play basketball and ride four-wheelers with a boyfriend. I think our classmates thought of us as boyfriend and girlfriend, but it was an unconventional relationship. Our activities were more like those of two good friends. We mostly played pickup basketball games with some other guys and rode Charles' four-wheeler.

I had wanted my own four-wheeler for a while, but I had never managed to buy one or talk my parents into buying one. I had been saving up my money to buy one when the "trouble" with the pistol occurred. Fixing that wiped out every penny I had saved. I wanted a four-wheeler more than anything, so I was always thrilled to go riding with Charles.

No Fear

On some occasions we would go all day with his family. I really looked forward to those times, and I so enjoyed riding.

After school, Charles would ride his four-wheeler to my house for our afternoon games of basketball. I had an adjustable goal, so we were all able to dunk and do things we couldn't do on a regulation-size goal. We spent hours and hours playing basketball. We would play rain or shine. When we weren't playing basketball, we rode the four-wheeler.

There were a few places around our houses for us to ride. For instance, we had permission from some neighbors to ride on their property. Covered with trails and hilly terrain, this spacious land was perfect for our adventures. Most of the time Charles' cousin Sean would go along with us.

One September day we were out riding with Sean. Charles and I were on one four-wheeler and Sean was on another. We set out for the neighbor's property. On one part of the property was a small rise that stood about two or three feet at a forty-five-degree angle. Charles and Sean were jumping the four-wheelers over the rise. They would back away from it, pick up speed, and hit it with the four-wheeler. When we hit it just right, we would fly through the air—at least it felt like we were flying. It got the adrenaline pumping and was a lot of fun. We had jumped this small hill three or four times when Charles pulled to a stop.

"Do you want to drive?" he asked.

"Yes, I'd love to," I replied.

I'd been hoping he would ask me this exact question, and I was elated when he finally did. We switched spots and were off again. At first I took it easy. It wasn't my four-wheeler, and I didn't feel comfortable going very fast yet. We rode around on the flat parts of the land, and I stayed away from anything very dangerous. I kept my cool and didn't push the four-wheeler too hard or too fast.

"Why don't you try jumping that hill?" Charles asked.

"Are you sure?" I replied, not wanting to appear too eager.

"Yeah, go ahead."

"Okay," I agreed.

I wasn't going to pass up an opportunity like this. I wasn't so sure I was ready to try the hill, but Charles seemed to think it was a good idea. He was an experienced driver, and I had his blessing. I was a little fearful, but I was not going to let fear stop me. If he was game, then I was game, so we started driving back away from the little hill so I could pick up enough speed to jump it.

No Fear

I lined up the four-wheeler with the hill and stomped on the gas. Who needs wise decisions? I was going to try this. We quickly gained speed, and the hill was getting closer and closer. Butterflies danced in my stomach, and I braced for the impact. We hit the little hill, caught air, and began to turn sideways on the four-wheeler. We were spinning through the air instead of staying upright. I had somehow managed to flip the four-wheeler when we jumped the hill!

If you've ever been in a wreck, you'll know what I mean when I say that everything around you seems like it happens in slow motion. We were getting viciously knocked around with every motion, yet while we flipped through the air time stood still. My body went one direction, Charles' went another direction, and the four-wheeler rolled along a separate trajectory. It was crazy. I just wanted everything to stop. Eventually the four-wheeler did stop and so did its former occupants.

It took me a few seconds to regain my thoughts. Still stunned, I looked around at Charles. He seemed to be okay, but he hadn't gotten up yet.

"Are you all right?" he asked.

"I think so," I said.

As Charles started to get up, I saw that he was holding his right arm close to his body. He only used his left arm to get off the ground, and he was not moving his right arm at all. I knew this couldn't be good. By then, Sean had returned to check on us.

"Are you guys okay?" he asked anxiously.

I nodded my head, still in some shock.

"I think something is wrong with my arm," Charles said.

"Can you drive?" asked Sean.

"I think so," Charles said.

"We need to get you guys some help," Sean said.

Charles and I slowly got back on the four-wheeler and headed for my house, which was only a mile away. We drove slower than we ever had, and Sean followed. Charles was driving with one arm, and that was a challenge on its own since the gas for the four-wheeler was on the handlebar. We slowly made our way back to my house. My mom was looking out her kitchen window wondering where we were when she saw us driving back. When she saw us driving so slowly, she knew something was wrong. Charles pulled into my drive, and I ran inside the house and told my mom what had happened.

Charles managed to make it back to his house, about a mile or so from my own house. I didn't go into detail at the time about how we had wrecked. I knew there would be plenty of time for that down the road, maybe when I turned eighteen. Minutes after I got home, Charles and his family went flying by our house on the way to the emergency room. We were worried about him and unsure of how bad his arm was.

Charles' arm was broken and required surgery. The doctors had to put a screw in his arm to repair it. I felt awful. I couldn't apologize enough to him. As a result of his injury, Charles missed part of that basketball season. Even though his arm healed, I knocked him out of many activities by deciding to try the jump. Charles was great about the whole thing and never seemed angry with me. I was blessed that he handled everything so gracefully. He and his family were wonderful to me as I learned another valuable lesson. It's unfortunate that they had to be involved in one of the lessons learned in my life.

Chapter 19

Happy Birthday to Me

On July 2, almost five months after my surgery, Dr. Wood released me. I arrived at the hospital at 3:40 p.m. to get a set of X-rays. After the X-rays were taken I headed down the hall to Dr. Wood's office. Justin and I sat in the waiting room in anticipation of meeting with him. I held to the optimistic expectation that he would say my back was doing well and I was free to do as I pleased. Although my hopes were high, I also feared he might say some part of my back did not look like it was healing properly and my freedom would be delayed. I was called back to a room and anxiously awaited his arrival.

"How have you been doing?" Dr. Wood asked as he entered my room.

"So-so I guess," I replied as I shrugged my shoulders. "I've been having some pain."

"I thought you might be dealing with that. Most people do at this stage," he said.

"How long will I continue to have pain?"

"We can't be sure, but some people have pain for twelve months."

It was normal? What a relief! When the pain had begun a few weeks before, I was crushed. I started thinking I had gone through all this for nothing. It was a devastating thought, and I became consumed with the fear of a life filled with pain. I would find solitude and break down in tears. Thus, Dr. Wood's words were like a ray of sunshine filling my mind and body with relief, hope, and joy.

Dr. Wood pulled up my X-rays on the computer and examined them.

"Everything looks real good," he said.

I beamed. "So can I do anything I want to now?"

"Yes," he said.

"Can I even lift things?"

As soon as I finished my question, Justin elaborated: "She wants to know if she can lift her brother."

"Does he have a disability?" Dr. Wood asked.

"Yes," I said. "He has cerebral palsy. He weighs about seventy pounds."

I could tell by the look on his face that he wasn't sure this was a good idea. You could see that he was thinking this question through before answering me. After a few seconds, he told me it would be okay.

This was a highly anticipated milestone. It was very exciting for me to hear that I could lift my brother again. As I previously mentioned, Christian requires a lot of care from my family. I help my parents when I can. Not being able to care for my brother had been one of the most difficult challenges I faced in my recovery. When Christian and my parents came to visit me, I got very frustrated because I could not hold him. I love this kid. He is wonderful and a joy for me to be around. I truly enjoy his company. On the day before my surgery, I made sure I carried him and cuddled him as much as possible. Now I would be able to pick him up and hold him again. I couldn't wait! I had waited a long time for this.

I also looked forward to resuming our bedtime ritual. When I'm at my parents' and Christian is going to bed, I stomp loudly through the house. Then I pick him up and carry him to bed. When he hears me coming, he gets so excited.

He really enjoys his sleep. Now, after almost five months, I would be able to enjoy this with him again.

The next day, July 3, was my birthday. The release from Dr. Wood had been the perfect gift for me. It was a good day, as I spent time with family. Justin met me at Best Buy and bought me an iPod, a wonderful gift. I am a music fanatic and loved the present. Then Justin and my mother-in-law, June, took me out for lunch in Bowling Green. We ate a delicious Japanese meal. When we got home the most wonderful thing happened to me. We had been mowing the yard that day, and I decided to try my back at using our weed-eater. I had not used it since the surgery.

"You don't need to be doing that," Justin said

"Dr. Wood released me. I have to start doing something sometime," I said.

I knew Justin was being protective, but I felt like I was ready. He made it clear he did not want me using the weed-eater, but I knew it was time to try. Justin was angry with me so he went inside our house. I don't really know if he was mad or if he couldn't watch. He had seen what bad shape I had been in, so this was probably hard for him. He might have even thought I couldn't start the weed-eater without him. He would have been right, but I asked June to start the weed-eater, and then I headed toward the yard with a big smile on my face.

I started around the house and got that done. Everything was going well, so I headed toward our pond. I walked with my shoulders back and my head held high. I felt a sense of pride at my accomplishment. I thought about how far I had come. Then I remembered everything I went through in the hospital—the surgery, the bedpans, the hospital gowns—and my pride deflated and my shoulders slumped a little. Who needs pride anyway? I had left mine at the hospital.

I walked around the pond, celebrating every weed I whacked. Yes! It was exhilarating to be able to do something like this again. I was overjoyed with weed-eating and so grateful to God for His healing touch. It sounds crazy to be elated with weed-eating, but I remembered those agonizing weeks of recovery: unable to get off the couch by myself, needing help up the steps, unable to get into bed on my own. Not long ago I couldn't even walk to the pond; now I was weed-eating the pond. Yes, at this stage in my life it did not take much to get me excited. As I walked around the pond, I sang "Amazing Grace" at the top of my lungs and worshipped God in the most unusual way. I was thankful for that weed-eater motor, which was loud enough to drown out the sound of my voice. More than anything, I was so grateful for how far God had brought me.

Chapter 20

Humbled

My surgery and recovery were a challenge. Each new day brought its own new fears. I battled fears I never thought would affect my life. The moment I agreed to do surgery, the fears started. I thought about the chance that I might not make it through the surgery. I was filled with dread when I pondered the recovery. I was afraid I might fall as I learned to walk again, and I was afraid of needles. As I listened to Dr. Wood talk about the pain, I was overcome with anxiety. I wondered all the time if I would ever be significant again. Would I be able to do anything that mattered? I doubted that I could find a place in life without the basketball skills I once knew. With my athleticism and strength gone, what would others see in me? What value would I have in this world?

The days before my surgery were filled with fear of not making it through the surgery. I looked at family and friends as if I might not see them again. I looked at God's beautiful landscapes with new eyes and new appreciation. I often questioned whether I was making the right decision. As the time grew closer, God comforted me with His presence and peace. Whenever I thought about not seeing tomorrow or the next day, I remembered where I would be if I weren't here on this earth. I knew I would be in heaven, and that thought granted me overwhelming peace and comfort.

Lying in the hospital, sometimes anxiety flooded me. As I said before, every morning when the tech came in to draw my blood my heart sank and tears filled my eyes. During my hospital stay I also became afraid of falling. I never felt safe with the small physical therapist as my safety net. What if I fell and messed up my back again? What if I had to go back into another surgery? My mind ran wild with dreadful thoughts and fears, but as always God gave me the courage to persevere. He gave me strength when I needed it, comfort when I needed it. He held me and carried me through each doubt and fear. "The Lord is my rock, my fortress and my deliverer; my God is my rock, in whom I take refuge" (Psalm 18:2 NIV).

My thoughts about the recovery were overwhelming. I couldn't imagine being off work for three months, not to mention being on the couch for six weeks. After the surgery, as I lay there on the couch staring at the ceiling, I didn't know if I could go on. I would feel sadness slowly creeping in. I didn't know if I could face another day immobilized. It was so hard to depend on others for everything. I couldn't even use the bathroom on my own! How do you find worth in your life like this? How do you find motivation to go on? How do you get yourself out of bed to face another mundane day? God was my hope and my motivation. As I lay there, He became more real to me than ever before. I was humbled before Him and quiet. Because I couldn't move a lot or didn't feel like talking, the door was opened for me to hear God and feel His presence even more. I was broken and battered, but He became strong for me. "For when I am weak, then I am strong" (2 Corinthians 12:10 NIV). It was the most uplifting feeling to be so dependent on God and to know that no matter how weak I was, He was all-powerful.

Pain filled each of my days for the first few weeks. The second day after the surgery I hurt so badly I didn't think I could make it. I pleaded for mercy and help, vocally and silently. I feared that the pain would overtake me mentally if it continued like it was. God granted His mercy, answering my prayers. When I thought I couldn't go on, God provided. He always does. With each challenge I faced, He was right there with me.

I got stronger each day, but I wondered if my life would ever be significant again. I was known as a basketball player. Often when people see me they say, "You must be a basketball player." I had never had an identity apart from basketball, but now I was going to have to face that. My skills were gone. My life would change. I didn't like this. I loved playing basketball, and I wasn't ready to put that behind me. What would people think of me if I couldn't dribble or shoot a ball anymore? Would I still matter to people? Would my life have any meaning? All I knew was playing, and now that was over for good. This was so hard to face. I couldn't see a future for myself because I didn't know what I would do.

As I recovered, I prayed, I studied, and I read often. As I took in God's Word and read other books, it became clear to me that my significance is not from a ball or from being able to jump high. My significance and your significance are the same. We are significant because we are children of God. I am His child. I have purpose in my life because of this. It doesn't matter what others think of me or what I can or can't do. I am important because God is my Father. I am so thankful that losing my abilities doesn't mean losing my life.

I am a different person now, but God can still use me. At the time of this writing, it has been six months since my surgery, but I still have to hold onto something when I bend over. I was strong, now I am weak. I was athletic, now I am clumsy. I am not the person I once was, but praise God that does not determine my value in life. I have been through so much, but I am grateful for how far God has brought me. I would not want to go through the surgery again, but God blessed me more than I could ever have imagined, and I am grateful for what I learned.

I saw God in a way I never had before, and it was amazing. I am thankful that I was so humbled and broken. The weaker I became, the stronger God became in my life. It taught me that I am not in control, God is. It felt good to let God take over and to rest in His arms. He brought me through so much and showed me so many things. I had to let go of what I knew and of the fears I faced and rely on His wonderful, merciful grace. I could feel His presence, and I could rely on His strength. It was the most wonderful thing to see God as I never had before. "My grace is sufficient for you, for my power is made perfect in weakness" (2 Corinthians 12:9 NIV).

Chapter 21

No Fear

Fear is everywhere. It is all around us—quiet yet overwhelming, silent yet demanding. Fear can imprison and immobilize its victims, affecting their work, relationships, and spiritual journey. It can overtake us. Fear, in some way or another, affects most of our lives. It whittles away our freedom and we may not even know it. We may fear death, failure, and sickness in addition to our fears of what others think about us. We fear rejection and judgment. Clearly, fear is a dominant force in our world and lives today.

I struggle with fear. I hate to write those words, but it's true. I fear losing my family. I fear being hurt by others, and I fear judgment of others. These fears sometimes direct my paths when they should not. Because of past hurts, I develop no new relationships. I am afraid others will also hurt me.

I try to protect myself from experiencing pain again. I tell myself as long as I don't have relationships with people, I can't get hurt. I have been so badly hurt in the past, and I don't want to feel that way again.

I am a very guarded person because of fear. As I write these words, I fear judgment and criticism from others. I write these things as one who struggles with you. I don't have all the answers, but I know who does: my Lord and God. I really believe this, and this belief is what gets me through. God, not fear, should direct my course and my choices. I should develop new friendships and relationships with others. I believe I miss out on God's blessings because I let fear guide me. "Two are better than one, because they have a good return for their work: If one falls down, his friend can help him up. But pity the man who falls and has no one to help him up!" (Ecclesiastes 4:9-10 NIV).

There are also times when I don't tell others about Jesus because I'm afraid of what they will think of me. I fear being judged. It is a privilege to have the opportunity to tell others about Jesus. It is a gift. Instead of focusing on the gift, I let the fear of rejection creep in. As a result, I miss the wonderful opportunity to spread the love of Christ. How many more people would know Jesus if we all put that fear behind us? To know Jesus is the most amazing relationship any of us can have, so why don't we spread His Word more?

I know my life would be different if I didn't allow myself to be affected by fear. My prayer is that I would allow the power of Jesus to operate in my life so I can defeat fear and move forward. I pray I would be able to leave the hurts of my past behind and step into the future with the hand of my Lord leading me. I want to trust Him and follow Him, kicking fear to the curb. I believe this is the path for living a life that's pleasing to the Lord, and that is what I want to do. Peace and joy follow a life that pleases God. Fear and troubles will arise, but God is more than these. He will take care of us and protect us. "I will say of the Lord, 'He is my refuge and my fortress, my God, in whom I trust'" (Psalm 91:2 NIV).

When I think about my childhood, I don't defend the things I did. I don't have pride in some of my choices. I did, however, confront fear. I did not back down. I did not run away. I challenged fear head-on and overcame it. Were my choices immature? Yes, clearly. I'm not saying we should drink perfume or jump off church balconies, but what if we step out into the world with that same reckless abandon? Without that fear, how many more people would we tell about Christ? How many more would we lead to Christ? I believe the numbers would be staggering.

Some fear is necessary to keep us from making impulsive, reckless decisions. Healthy fear, coupled with godly wisdom, make a great combination. It is when we let fear stop us from following the Lord that it becomes detrimental. When fear runs our life in a negative way, it is of no benefit. However, righteous fear, or reverence for God, brings Him glory. In fact, God's Word says that the fear of the Lord is the beginning of wisdom. "The fear of the Lord is the beginning of knowledge, but fools despise wisdom and discipline" (Proverbs 1:7 NIV).

If you have these struggles, you are not alone. You are far from alone. I struggle with you and so do others. Many may not even recognize it for what it really is. I pray we would all lift up our voices to the Lord; He will hear our call. He will hold us and strengthen us and cast out our fears. "There is no fear in love, but perfect love casts out fear" (1 John 4:18 NKJV).

God has a plan for each and every one of us. We can trust Him and look to Him for the wonderful blessings He has for us now and in the days ahead. He tells us that in His Word.

"There is hope in your future, says the Lord" (Jeremiah 31:17 NKJV).

We may not be able to explain everything that happens. Who can explain a sick child or the good person who develops cancer? I know I can't. I think sometimes this adds to our fears because we strongly desire to have control. It doesn't matter how much we fear something or worry about something, we can't change certain things. We should try to change the things we can. We can change our actions and stop letting fear drive us. We can pray for fear to leave us so that we may stand up for the Lord and for things that are important to us. With things we can't change, we must leave them to God and trust Him. "Trust in the Lord with all your heart and lean not on your own understanding" (Proverbs 3:5 NIV).

I desire to live my life without fear, like my childhood self. I want to run forward, following my Lord. He alone is in control. He is the God who overcomes fear. He is alive and with us each and every day. It is not a coincidence that the phase "fear not" appears in the Bible 365 times. I had the privilege of facing fears, being broken, and watching God work in a special way in my life. Because of those challenges, God seemed closer to me than ever before. The time

I spent feeling broken and battered, I would not trade for anything. I am thankful for God strengthening me and being so real to me during that time. I am thankful He allowed me to go through what I did so I could become closer to Him. I was never alone, and you are not alone.

Our God is a mighty God who can overcome any fear we have. If we keep our focus on Him, our fears will fade away. The Lord guided me through all the fears I faced, and He will guide you. He is the almighty, powerful God. "I sought the Lord, and he answered me; he delivered me from all my fears" (Psalm 34:4 NIV).

LaVergne, TN USA
29 December 2010
210445LV00003B/133/P